Perspectives on Dentistry

An Insider's Guide to the Professional Business of Dental Hygiene

DEBORAH STEWART, RDH, MBA, PCC

Perspectives on Dentistry
An Insider's Guide to the Professional Business of Dental Hygiene
© 2014 Deborah Stewart

Disclaimer: These perspectives on dentistry are solely those of the author based on 45 years of experience as a dental hygienist in the State of Texas and deep knowledge of the field of dentistry in general.

Author: Deborah Stewart
Editor: Barbara McNichol Editorial
Cover: CreateSpace
Interior Design: Peggy Henrikson

Manufactured in the United States of America

First printing, March 2014

ISBN-10: 1492206954
ISBN-13: 978-1492206958

CONTENTS

DEDICATION

This book is dedicated to the memory of Dona Arnold Myers, 1950-2013, my roommate at Texas Woman's University.

Dona worked as a dental hygienist in Dallas, Texas, for over 35 years and was an active member of the American Dental Hygienists Association. Her roommates Nancy Brooks, Joan Edwards Harkin, and I called her "the General" because she represented the best of dental hygiene skills and leadership. A caring human being, Dona dedicated herself to helping those who were lucky enough to be her friends. After meeting and working with Dona, one emerged not only with more proficient dental skills but wiser, with better character because, like a good general, she could inspire the best in others.

ACKNOWLEDGMENTS

My parents, Chris and Ann Perry, have always encouraged education. Their support of learning and their reflection in my life were gifts of unconditional love.

My children, Todd and Meagan, have allowed me to fuss and fret over their teeth and teach them about dentistry. Todd Stewart is a physician and emergency room resident in San Antonio, Texas. The field of medicine is a perfect fit for Todd because of his relaxed personality, decision-making abilities, and patience. Meagan is a dietitian and physician assistant in lap band surgery and obesity.

One day when Meagan was in third grade, I came home from work and was preparing dinner only to find her eating cake and candy. I immediately discarded the junk food in the kitchen because, as a mother and dental hygienist, I needed to provide healthy foods. Meagan credits her decision to become a dietitian to that event. Hers is another example of changed perceptions allowing growth, intuition, and behavioral direction.

I am honored to be Todd and Meagan's mother, not because of what they have chosen as professions, but who they are inside. They have been a great source of love and energy to me. God has blessed me with a wonderful family, including a grandson and son-in-law to love, as well as friends who seem like family to me.

What good fortune and honor I received to be taught by Dr. Nancy Glick, teacher emeritus and mentor at Texas Woman's University. Dr. Glick willed me her strength at times much like the visually symbolized pioneer woman statue at TWU in Denton, Texas. The pioneer woman statue is 15 feet tall and made of Georgian white marble. It was sculpted by New York City artist Leo Friedlander. Unveiled in 1938 in honor of the Texas Centennial, the statue stands as a tribute to the spirit of the pioneer women of Texas. Walking by the statue is inspirational, but conversations with Dr. Glick would stimulate my mind to a higher level of activity, and many years after graduation, those conversations continue to do so.

I greatly appreciate the professors at the University of Texas at Dallas, who were always positive in their affirmations. My heart expresses thanks to Dr. Robert Hicks, Judy Feld, and Judy Clothier for the caring hands that continue to lift me up and push me forward. Teachers who inspire provide persuasive logic because the best move is sometimes a bold move.

A special thank you goes to Beth Sparks and Matthew Dann, who provide financial advice at Wells Fargo Advisors, and Barbara McNichol, who edited this book.

Thank you to all who endure my idiosyncrasies and discussions concerning the business of dentistry. Friends who share their perspectives, add thoughtful reflections, and help translate the vision into real-world outcomes are indispensable to me in navigating this "road trip" of my career.

MESSAGE FROM DEBORAH

"I slept and dreamt that life was joy. I awoke and saw that life was service. I acted and behold, service was joy."

– Rabindranath Tagore

To future students who choose dentistry as a profession: Study hard, learn from your teachers, expand your scope of practice, and realize what an honor it is to be a healthcare provider. Never take the dental profession for granted. Dentistry can be a most fulfilling, rewarding, and giving profession by helping co-workers find fulfillment in their work, helping them succeed, and improving the quality of life for patients.

I sincerely hope this book *Perspectives on Dentistry: An Insider's Guide to the Professional Business of Dental Hygiene* serves as a reminder of the profound impact dentistry can create, an endeavor that, managed correctly by leadership, is nothing short of a gift from God.

– Deborah Lynn Malone Stewart

PREFACE

"Never, never give up."

– Winston Churchill

It's difficult for me to believe that the profession of dental hygiene is more than 100 years old. What would the dental profession have been without the contribution of Dr. Alfred Civilion Fones? As a dentist in the early 1900s, Dr. Fones was concerned about the number of patients losing their teeth due to dental caries and periodontal disease. Convinced that the removal of plaque and calculus from the surfaces of the teeth and gingival margins could reduce or prevent tooth loss, he began a crusade to persuade others in the dental and medical fields that some dental diseases could be prevented.

In 1906, without support from many health professionals, Dr. Fones trained Irene Newman to be the first dental hygienist in the world. Her purpose was to provide preventive dental cleanings to his patients. The results were so successful that he spent much of his time during the next years spreading the word about the new member of the dental team. In 1913, he opened the Fones School of Dental Hygiene in Bridgeport, Connecticut.

Dr. Fones certainly had an inspired vision. His philosophy of teaching dental disease prevention has been the most important development in the history of dentistry. Connecticut is considered the birthplace of dental hygiene and the Fones School a model for advanced progressive education. The newly developed Advanced Practice Dental Hygienist (APDH) degree program is a testimony to the visionary Dr. Fones.

In Texas, the state where I live and work, dental hygienists are employed by the dentist in private practice versus corporate dentistry and public health clinics, in which the salary is paid by the organization. Although each facility of employment has a basic code of ethics, hygienists have their own code of ethics and practice values, and the public has come to trust these values. They include helping the public maintain optimal oral health, nutritional counseling, and oral cancer education as well as applying cavity-preventive material to teeth.

Dental hygienists focus on preventive care and motivate others to do their best. People want to be around such positive energy. Healthcare professionals who focus on the positive aspect of health usually have a higher percentage of patient adherence to a recommended course of treatment. This gives dental hygienists a leadership advantage because patients believe in and easily accept the treatment presented. A higher rate of treatment acceptance reinforces confidence in dental hygiene professionals. As a result, hygienists desire to expand duties, which is why I believe a disconnect with the dentist occurs at critical points.

When there is more patient acceptance, then hygienists want to improve and expand their dental skills. As technologies improve, dental hygienists want to apply newly learned skills. If some of these skills are ones that only the dentist performs, then friction concerning boundaries can erupt. The area of periodontics is an area of expanding technologies. For hygienists, laser treatments for periodontal disease will routinely become an area of shared responsibility with the dentist, needing the goodwill of hygienists to trust and explain complex treatments to patients.

No job is perfect, and the profession of dental hygiene is not without stress. Working in the dental industry takes commitment, dedication, and continued learning. Today's dentists and dental hygienists face many more issues than ever before imagined. However, the rewards are clear: Hygienists are giving people a more confident dental experience and enhancing their health, while working with people who share a passion for the profession.

Purpose of This Book

This book has been written to encourage and inspire dental hygienists to become leaders in the field of dentistry. As a hygienist, you can become more aware of your business environment and develop the skills to improve working conditions not only for your team members but for your patients.

In addition, you can learn to guard your ethics—because change and challenges present themselves every day. This book addresses the many issues you'll face, providing information you need to know to be successful in your career. These issues include:

- Professionalism in dentistry

- Technology changes

- Role of hygienists in relation to dentists

- Ethics in dentistry

- A supportive business culture

- Progression of professional organizations

I hope that by sharing what I've learned throughout my journey as a dental hygienist, you will save time and avert potential problems. This book provides possible directions for your own path.

INTRODUCTION: EMBARKING ON YOUR JOURNEY IN DENTISTRY

"You can't cross the sea merely by standing and staring at the water."

– Rabindranath Tagore

The study and practice of dental hygiene is like taking a road trip. That is, you decide where you're going and who you wish to take on the journey.

Here's the image I have kept in my mind over the years to help me embrace changes along my career journey: I have a map and my car is in good working order. I learn the landmarks and seek to make informed decisions while enjoying the drive. I have reasonable expectations about the daily drive to achieve my destination. I keep at a controlled speed and watch carefully for warning signs that I'm not speeding. I avoid disrespectful drivers, but if they bump into me, I repair the damage quickly and move on.

A license to practice the dental hygiene profession is your opportunity to get in the car and begin an adventurous road trip. Like driving a car, I've always considered this career to be a privilege as well as an opportunity. Why is it an opportunity? Because forming the right skills, alliances, and practices can lead to incredible advances in learning—and great career satisfaction for you.

To Make the Best of Your Career

Striving to be what you imagine—envisioning your destinations along the way—can help you manifest what you want. Therefore, as you start your career journey, make sure you associate with experienced hygienists who can critique your services. I suggest actively seeking practicing hygienists who have exceptionally good clinical skills. To succeed, imitate and model their values. Invite communication that leads to enhanced skill-building and continually ask to be mentored.

Making the best of this career also requires being accountable yourself, demanding accountability from others, and being coachable when crossroad decisions or changes are necessary. Learning new technologies and techniques will improve the level of your skills and add to the scope of services you can provide.

Preparing for Your Career's "Road Trip"

Mapping out your role in this profession will help you navigate through your day. Just as you'd list the top things you'd do to prepare for your road trip, making a list can make your career journey as smooth as possible. Consider these requirements:

- Develop strong oral hygiene instruction skills.

- Be highly observant and embrace agility, change, and speed.

- Learn your profession well and quickly, making sure it aligns with your core values.

- Develop grit as you realize those achievements.

- Read dental and dental hygiene magazines to keep up to date on the latest trends.

- Perform dental hygiene services on or with experienced hygienists to gain mastery.

- Organize a study club with dentists and hygienists to discuss unique cases and critique dental hygiene business models for their efficiency.

- Volunteer to present programs about skills you know at professional meetings.

- Study specific protocols for attracting new patients and retaining existing patients.

- Learn the demographics of your practice location and engage with the community of people you serve.

- Show active listening skills, even restating what the speaker is saying to ensure your proper understanding.

- Bring people together often for positive talks, including the patient and the dentist.

- Take advantage of being evaluated by those who already have the service tools of the profession—because learning is ongoing and lasts a lifetime.

Interpersonal and Behavioral Skills Top the List

In a professional clinical setting, oral hygiene instruction (OHI), which refers to teaching and motivating patients, is perhaps the most important skill to learn. Unfortunately, because billable time for OHI isn't typically covered by insurance, it's often overlooked in dental offices. The hygienist sees the patient every three to six months, but health care at home is important to do every day. Many hygienists remind patients by newsletters, blogs, and social media to stay connected, establish a professional relationship, and gain the trust of patients.

Because dental hygiene is a profession based on teaching and technical skills rather than a business based on commodities and products, relating behaviors to business productivity might be questioned. Yet developing strong personal relationships is an important part of delivering healthcare. After all, communication, professionalism, gratitude, leadership, and ethics all intersect at the point of behavior—for all professionals including hygienists.

To adopt desired behaviors, again, you're wise to connect to positive people who will influence you in ways you don't even realize. For example, to quit smoking, smokers make new friends who do not smoke. Naturally, these friends will enforce a no-smoking rule.

What to Expect Going Forward

Behaviors are contagious, and when enough people change a behavior, it often becomes the norm. By carefully reading this book, you can expect to learn:

- How to take ownership of sustainable growth in your dental hygiene department.

- Why developing a budget is important.

- How to nurture a collegial partnership with the dentist you work with.

- Why having your own retirement plan separate from the dentist's plan is critical.

As you explore the chapters that follow, I know you'll find a way to map out your personal road trip. Have fun as you imagine your journey and reach the destination of your dreams.

CHAPTER 1: WHERE IS THE DENTAL INDUSTRY HEADED?

"Action indeed is the sole medium of expression for ethics."

— Jane Addams

Actions have always spoken louder than words, especially in the dental field. Having observed relationships between dentists and dental hygienists over a 45-year professional career, I believe our industry may be heading the wrong way.

For example, the increase in Medicaid fraud by dentists leads to mistrust by the public. Dentists set the "tone at the top." When cases of dental fraud are reported by the television news stations, the public questions whether those in the dental industry are putting the needs of their patients first. How does the hygienist model exceptional care when there's a degree of skepticism within the public regarding the overall profession?

Second, the team knows if the dentist is committed to comprehensive care, so how do you overlook deception and market the practice if you are unsure that the poor behavior will not happen to you? The inability to expand duties for dental hygienists leads to underutilizing skills and stagnation of the profession. As a hygienist, do you feel frustration about the progression of the dental hygiene industry? Have poor working relationships between dentists and hygienists added friction in your experience?

As dental hygienists, we must be our own advocates, and we face a few issues.

Issues Hygienists Face

First of all, the sheer dominance of technology is an integral part of performing your clinical skills. Integrating social media that includes the best ways to remind patients of appointments can be overwhelming. Sure, the principles of oral hygiene are taught in schools, but how do you prepare for the multitude of sales presentations with new products, learn new office software, and develop accurate ways of recording chart notes while operating in a daily time crunch? How do you deal with the stress of recently mastered digital radiology and the dentist in charge determines the team must learn cone beam CT scans? How do you integrate laser periodontal therapy into the practice? These new technologies will be part of your responsibilities, so how can you master the competencies technology demands and not be overwhelmed?

Second, external and internal limitations hinder on-the-job development. For example, several states allow hygienists to have independent practice while 45 states allow hygienists to perform local anesthesia. But this is not so in Texas where I live. In Texas, dental hygienists are required to work under the indirect supervision of a dentist. Advanced dental hygiene practitioner programs that exist in other states are not offered in Texas. As a result, hygienists with advanced skills who relocate to Texas from other states have more opportunities to find employment, especially in education. Certainly one thing the dental industry needs is advanced trained dental hygienists to join the public health team. Expanding clinical opportunities to help disabled population groups, children, and the elderly could improve quality of life and employment opportunities for dental hygienists in Texas hospitals, nursing homes, and schools.

Third, confusion comes when Texas dentists consider hygienists to be independent contractors when it comes to compensation, but IRS "Guidelines for Employee versus Independent Contractor" classify the vast majority of hygienists as employees. Therefore, the independent classification could be regarded as an unlawful employer tax dodge. As a consequence, hygienists whose offices don't report their compensation to the Texas Workforce Commission (TWC) and pay TWC taxes wouldn't be eligible for unemployment compensation.

Fourth, when hygienists are paid as contractors, they are responsible for withholding their own federal income tax and social security tax. In fact, they must pay double the social security tax because, in a normal pay situation, employers match that tax for the employee. Because the dental hygienist is considered an employee of the dentist under Texas state and federal law, if dentists don't pay these taxes, they're subject to IRS and TWC audits and penalties. Both dentists and hygienists need to be aware of this situation.

Working Interviews

Confusion may be compounded by employment agencies that provide "working interviews." During the interview time, the dentist observes the skills of a recent graduate over a day or a week before permanently hiring the individual. So-called "working interviews" aren't lawful under every state's labor laws and can constitute an initiation of employment. Working for free is not an option unless the hygienist is in the office only to observe.

A myriad of problems can arise in this situation:

- What happens when the candidate is presented a daily schedule that seriously impacts the dentist's schedule? Is there time for advanced preparation?

- Is a typical one-day or one-week working interview really an indication of what the applicant and practice have to offer each other?

- What happens if a candidate on a working interview is stuck with an infected needle or injured at the office? Is there insurance coverage for such an event?

- What happens if the candidate breaks a piece of equipment? Who is responsible for repairs?

- How will the office ensure that a working-interview non-employee will follow HIPAA regulations?

Working interviews are a challenge to the credibility of the office. Hygienists who work temporary jobs do not achieve retirement goals. In addition, long-term continuing education, exposure to technology, and extended learning as a valuable member of the team are never realized.

If a practice benefits financially from the work of another person, labor laws state that the person must be compensated. Therefore, a contract between dentist and dental hygienist is required to address questions that might affect employment.

The best way to hire is to conduct proper interviews and check references. Candidates must do their own due diligence to check references on the practice and ask key questions during the interview. Nothing guarantees a successful working relationship for both dentist and hygienist, but taking precautions when beginning the process provides a good foundation.

Balancing Value and Cost

Typically, dental assistants work with the dentist on procedures that are billed by the dentist. Hygienists conduct procedures independent of the dentist in a separate workspace. Because of this separate workspace, it's important for hygienists to be aware of the costs to the practice for providing dental hygiene services.

What is the baseline cost to keep the dental practice open daily? Knowing this figure—plus the amount of profit that can be produced to offset it—helps a hygienist understand what percentage of the cost he or she is responsible for when considering salary. This knowledge can aid in reducing stress in the office and help build partnership with the dentist.

Calculating Costs

Hygienists can calculate their degree of obligation or expense as well as their contribution to total production in the office. Let's say the total rent of the office and supplies for the hygienist are $75,000 a year. What percentage of that rent and supplies does the dentist think the hygienist should contribute to calculate salary?

Do you see the benefit of knowing? Having an idea of the cost involved in performing the job will help engender communication concerning a hygienist's value to the practice. The business of dentistry includes shared skills, and sharing precise information can allow for more frequent salary increases for all members of the dental team.

CHAPTER 2: MY JOURNEY IN DENTISTRY—AND YOURS

"Treat people with respect, do no harm to patients, promote the well-being of the public, and accept responsibility to tell the truth."

– Deborah Stewart

In my first job as a dental assistant, I fell in love with dentistry. I was hired by Dr. Robert Kunkle, a man of wit similar to that of actor Walter Matthau. This seasoned dentist in Garland, Texas, taught me how to take radiographs and develop them perfectly. It was a summer job, and every day, Dr. Kunkle thought I wouldn't return, but I kept coming back so he could "lovingly" teach me. On my last day of working there, he encouraged me to apply to dental hygiene school—so I did.

As a hygienist, I worked for Dr. Tipton Asher, a pedodontist. A brilliant clinician and teacher, Dr. Asher knew everything there was to know about exfoliation of deciduous teeth. Before digital radiographs, he would place a Kodak panoramic x-ray on the viewer and ask me to diagnose the problem. He mentored me both personally and professionally, and I trusted his advice. I knew he had my best interests at heart.

In addition, I worked for Dr. Ed Bridgeman, a general dentist, who continued my mentoring and advanced my skill level—not only as a hygienist but as an office manager. Always starting the day with a smile and a joke, he lifted my understanding of quality of life while teaching me the business of dentistry. Determined that dentistry needed hygienists who had strong business skills, I attended the University of Houston and graduated with a Master of Business Administration.

The Changing Face of Dentistry

Here's how I have observed the changes in dentistry over the years. The service has evolved from a small office composed of a dentist, dental hygienist, and assistant with emphasis on preventive and restorative care to a cosmetic business focused on patient cases worth thousands of dollars. That focus lasted 20-plus years. What has now emerged is a corporate practice with multiple dental offices and a production mentality. That mentality was decided by owners and managers of the practice, not necessarily the dentists themselves.

Many questions arose: What problems would this new business approach cause within the dental hygienist industry? What research was available concerning multiple practice models? Did the head dentist manage the practice, or did multiple dentists with corporate thinking run the practice? I had to investigate what was happening and have been asking lots of questions.

What understanding was necessary to determine how dentists wanted their businesses to perform—and were their perceptions realistic? Were dentists still in charge of their own offices? My research indicated that often they were not, despite Texas law. Were business investments and hedge funds that invest in corporations changing the delivery of dental services?

In 2010, I seized the opportunity to attend the University of Texas at Dallas to study organizational behavior. This is the study of business activities involving achievement and economic realities to prevent practice disruptions. Could new business models provide new opportunities—and how would this affect the role of the dental hygienist? This book addresses many of these questions.

Dental graduates hired by corporate dental facilities need an immediate paycheck due to student loan debt and a need to increase their speed when performing dentistry. Because dentists get paid by procedure, in effect, they compete with hygienists for doing the procedure hygienists typically do. Chances are, no relationships are developed with hygienists in this setting. The dentist cleans the teeth, and the assistant polishes them. Hygienists therefore don't have professional relationships with corporate-employed dentists and miss out on the opportunity to provide long-term patient care.

The concept of corporate practice for hygienists is still in its formative years. The only thing I can compare it to is my time in public health but with this difference: *The concept of competition between employed dentist and hygienist changes the team concept of working together.* Ideally, the dentist should relinquish the prophylaxis dental procedure to the hygienist who is the most trained to perform this procedure. In my opinion, a business model that doesn't promote a collegial relationship between the team of dentists and hygienists will not advance the profession of hygiene nor will it provide excellent preventive care.

Of great concern to hygienists is the amount of investment money corporate dentistry can attract. Hedge funds invest in a dental company to make a profit or to buy the entity at a cheap price and provide investment returns for the original investors. If you work in the dental business, could hedge funds have negative implications for you as an employee? Know that the further away from ownership you work, the more "commodity like" your work becomes to the owner of the business. For hygienists, this means the relationships between patient and dentist will change, but you have the right and obligation to work safely.

No doubt you've seen how much corporate dentistry advertises on television. The ads promise to provide teeth restorations in a day. In our society, when television advertises successful surgical cases, then the public believes these procedures are safe. Oral surgeons, periodontists, and surgical assistants work side by side in facilities that have a surgical suite while in a neighboring room, the laboratory designs the denture or prosthetic device the same day.

Is this a more efficient way for specialists to practice? The specialists are employees paid by the corporation; they are no longer responsible for providing funding for the technology and the updates required. These facilities have become much like hospitals that provide one type of procedure, e.g., implants with prosthetic dentures. As long as the patient base requiring this one type of procedure continues to exist, then the investment is fairly risk free. Investment funding becomes available for these centers to buy technology that has been unavailable or out of reach for private practice, especially general dentists who practice solo.

The issue that these organizations are growing with equity money is important to understand. The door has been opened to lure investors, even dentists, who wish to invest in the business of corporate dentistry. The equity money used to invest, buy, or con-solidate private practices has increased. All this is having massive implications on the dental industry. It means with fewer private practices, the number of potential jobs for dental hygienists is reduced.

Basically, the typical solo dentist can only raise money through debt, but growing a practice rapidly through acquisition of debt is difficult. Given today's corporate dentistry environment, these questions must be asked:

- How will the use of hedge money to supply the capital affect the dental industry?

- Has the focus of providing preventive services as a team between general dentists and dental hygienists been disrupted?

- Are hygienists being constricted from corporate dental models because preventive service skills have a relatively low margin of profit?

- Is it more important to employ certain dentists because they possess restorative skills and can perform preventive skills with the aid of an assistant?

- Will this new model improve patients' oral healthcare?

What concerns do you have about the future of the profession of dental hygiene?

The Importance of Communication

One of the behaviors that's crucial to success is effective communication. Many in today's workforce grew up on video games, texting, and email, with little need to use full sentences by speaking directly to another person. The average 20 year old expects to change careers over five times in his or her lifetime. However, dentistry is a career that requires a lot of commitment of time and expertise.

Communicating well is a necessary skill for hygienists. Presenting dental treatment plans involves engaging fully with the patient to explain the plan. That's only one way hygienists are required to listen to their patients and communicate well. They also pay attention to nonverbal behaviors while presenting oral hygiene treatment, giving instructions, taking radiographs, and providing fluoride treatments.

Patients value a personalized relationship with "their" hygienist who expresses concern about their family and overall well-being. If a hygienist changes offices within a community, patients often change practices. They want to continue with that special person they know, value, and trust.

The ideal type of connection represents all of these qualities and techniques that promote the profession of dentistry well:

- Having a warm, friendly attitude, asking questions, and showing interest in patients

- Being a resource, providing logical approaches in answer to any questions

- Being knowledgeable about the dental industry

- Matching the patient with the best products as needed

- Networking with others to address issues beyond the scope of practice

Are Hygienists in the Business of Teeth or People?

We are in the people business. We're trained professionals trusted with the opportunity to provide oral health care. Good dental hygiene practitioners facilitate a partnership with each patient to attain and maintain optimal oral health. Therefore, training in interpersonal communication skills constitutes an integral part of the dental hygiene curriculum.

As a result, students who have a sufficient facility in English are able to:

- Obtain information from a variety of learning resources;

- Convey concepts and knowledge on written examinations;

- Elicit patient histories, problems, and symptoms;

- Record and retrieve information from patient charts; and

- Coordinate patient care with all members of the health care team.

As hygienists, we're taught to listen and look at the patient while asking questions, identify and process information, and develop part of the treatment plan after examination. When we perform our duties with an attractive smile and encourage others to reciprocate, we provide a model that inspires patients to become better educated about their oral hygiene. A smile helps make people more approachable. In turn, approachable people usually have better interpersonal skills, and better communication makes for a better world.

Interpersonal communication skills are vital to the practice of dentistry, much like skills used to diagnosis a medical or dental problem. If we ask a patient to value dentistry as preventive healthcare and maintain daily home care, then the practitioner must also commit time to improve clinical as well as interpersonal skills. We use these same diagnostic skills to constantly improve our own communication skills.

Overall, the goal is having a healthy patient. Knowledge and dental skills are important, but connecting with people and developing interpersonal skills makes a practice thrive. Continue reading and see how you can create a legacy for yourself in this profession.

CHAPTER 3: THE FORWARD-LOOKING ROLE OF HYGIENISTS

"All labor that uplifts humanity has dignity and importance and should be undertaken with painstaking excellence."

– Reverend Dr. Martin Luther King

The more skills you have—in dentistry, communication, or business—the more secure your career will be.

Statistics indicate that as more schools of dental hygiene form, the number of dental hygienists dramatically increases. In the North Texas area, the number of schools has doubled from three to six. Two schools offer completion of a degree in 18 months rather than four years. The curriculum seems ideal for community colleges, and the growth of public community college districts in Texas continues to grow—from 40 in 1968 to 50 in 1995.

Higher costs of education in four-year programs fuel the growth of community colleges with more students trying to receive an education. In 2010, two additional for-profit dental hygiene schools were formed with Stanford Brown and Concorde. This brings the total to six schools in the Dallas-Ft. Worth metro area. When you add Texas A&M Baylor College of Dentistry, Texas Woman's University, and Collin and Tarrant County colleges, the collective number exceeds 100 graduates yearly.

As more hygienists are graduated from these colleges, where will they find jobs if employment is restricted to working in a dentist's office?

In this same period, no new Texas dental schools have been accredited. Were student dentists being graduated at this increased rate or even a rate that will transition the practices of mature dentists? The recession of 2009 caused dentists to postpone retirement, and because the seasoned dentists continue to work, the dental industry is evolving around them. This new way of working may be stressful. Let's look at why.

Benefits for a dentist buying an existing practice have always included initial patient acceptance, instant practice organization, and a tenured team, but there are no guarantees. For example, if either of the dentists during the transition pressures the employees, including the dental hygienist, to sell more products or services to patients, then patients may become uncomfortable and leave the practice. Therefore, the hygienist needs to be an advocate for patients, working to ensure they feel comfortable with the care and not feel like they're always being up-sold. The hygienist also wants to feel confident during any transitions that the care given in the office is ethical and reflects updated research.

Change Requires Continual Learning

With a younger dentist to introduce new trends of periodontal awareness and add changes to the system, you can be vulnerable if you're not open to learning new systems and being adaptable in your skill level. Feeling attuned to another involves being attuned to yourself.

Although the dental hygiene profession has been taught for more than a century, change is constant. Continued learning requires development of harmonious and responsive relationships because improvements involve technology, materials, and techniques. Therefore, you're wise to volunteer and attend local educational programs, take advantage of classes including web-based continuing education courses, study clubs, and make learning a daily habit. Your desire to improve reinforces your leadership abilities.

Constantly Assess Job Markets for Hygienists

Estimates indicate that new graduates take an average of six months to one year to secure a job, but temporary jobs are available. You're wise to write a résumé and always have 20 copies in your possession at all times. After all, you never know when a conversation will provide an opportunity for follow-up.

In the North Texas area, more than 100 hygienists graduate yearly, so if you live in that area—or wherever you live—it's good to contract with several dental employment agencies. Associate-degreed hygienists are usually employed in a clinical practice by a dentist in private practice, public health, or corporate dentistry. Alternative employment of dental hygienists in sales, administrative jobs, and education require a bachelor's degree, and some teaching positions may require a master's degree.

The Texas Dental Association (TDA) and Texas Practice Act have granted dental assistants the opportunity to be trained in coronal polishing. In reality, a dentist can remove the calcified deposits on the teeth and allow the assistant to polish, thus reducing the need for hiring a hygienist. Unfortunately, there are dentists who allow assistants to unlawfully perform other services. (This information is described in detail on the websites of many state boards when researching complaints and disciplinary actions taken by the State Board of Dental Examiners.) Coronal polishing by assistants has added to the numbers of underemployed hygienists. Especially with a lower demand, it's important for hygienists to continue their education. Make sure your course work and degree are transferable to another college.

Generally, even seasoned private practice dentists can't subsidize a dental hygiene department. Dentists want the hours the hygienist is working to be productive; when there is unfilled appointment time, they expect hygienists to reduce their compensation or make the necessary changes to improve the schedule.

With seasoned dentists not retiring and fewer businesses providing dental insurance, dentists may decide to support their office overhead and themselves by reducing the number of employees. In a slow economy, the professionals most severely affected by such practices are dental hygienists, "the middle class" of the dental industry.

If you're a new dental hygiene graduate, it's important to associate with seasoned hygienists who are running profitable dental hygiene departments. Many business models exist, but most fall into three categories based on time spent with the patient:

- Dental hygienist working in one room with no assistant seeing an adult patient every hour and every half-hour for children.

- Dental hygienist working in two rooms seeing a patient every 30 minutes with an assistant performing auxiliary duties such as sterilization of instruments, cleaning the rooms between patients, taking radiographs, and fluoride treatments (total patient time of one hour).

- Dental hygienist working in one room with no assistant seeing a patient (adult, adolescent, child) every 30 minutes.

Adaptability to how the dentist or the corporation wants to structure the hygiene department is the key factor in job approval, so it's essential to know how you like to provide services. Job satisfaction depends on team-driven productivity that includes the hygienist and provides patients with better dental care. However, the practice has to establish a base to be able to pay the hygienist's salary and still make a profit.

Multiple Facilities and Care Providers

Some dental management companies promote models of employment with multiple facilities and multiple care providers. Large facilities have production incentives you must achieve. As a new graduate, you may find yourself in a position to join this type of environment in which production is the top priority. However, my experience suggests it's best to first find employment where you can have a mentor dentist or study group to help with the transition process. A hygienist is advised to never compromise patient-centered care for production.

Never once did my mentors make unreasonable demands, but at times, the goals were challenging. A hygienist may be asked by the dentist to see an adult patient in 30 to 45 minutes, so it's challenging not to sacrifice professionalism in a time period that usually takes one hour. Well-run offices set realistic goals that improve performance of clinical skills while increasing productivity. Well-defined goals that empower and provide greater retention of employees produce lower costs of operation. Constantly learning ways to work with other team members more efficiently has its rewards, especially in technology or skills improvement. Even if you have a permanent job, volunteering at a health fair or working in different dental offices keeps your skills current because you will learn from and be exposed to other professionals.

Statistics from a 2004 article by Dr. Eric Solomon in *Dental Economics* titled "The Future of Dentistry" indicate that, through the year 2020, there will be fewer dental graduates compared to older practitioners. Although dental students have been graduating at a constant rate for the last 10 to 12 years, in 2013, seasoned dentists outnumbered new dental graduates, especially in populated areas. The baby boom-aged dentists are retiring, but to prolong work, a trend has developed for seasoned dentists to form large group practices and have multiple office locations. What is the result? Having multiple offices increases overhead costs and puts stress on older clinicians to add production and staff, including hygienists and new dental graduates.

The model for facility growth in dental clinics has been largely due to several corporate dentistry companies that manage more than 300 dental clinics in 20 states and employ thousands of people. Dentistry is labeled as a cottage industry because its products are not mass produced. Private investor companies saw this as a weakness ripe for management services, which resulted in the growth of dental chains. The welfare of the patient is at the center of this controversy. Growth of this corporate dentistry concept has allowed two companies to be in the top 10 list of job creators in the United States, with each company adding over a thousand jobs.

Job Growth Doesn't Mean Job Happiness

Many graduating dentists and hygienists find employment in corporate dentistry, but this type of working environment doesn't necessarily translate to job happiness. Plus, geographical growth doesn't necessarily mean more people will come to the facility and become patients. Transitions require much thought at the beginning of a career and especially in the process of retiring.

One-office locations tend to allow the dentist and support team more opportunity and flexibility for educational growth compared with large group practices in multiple locations. My preferred employment opportunities have been with two dentists in one location so that if one dentist retires, the other dentist is in place to begin the transition process. It may take longer for older professionals to transition a new professional, but a longer transition time may be best for patients and team members in the office. This allows for an adjustment period for relationships to form, training to occur, and new strategies to be perfected.

During periods of adjustment, 7 to 10 percent of patients may leave a practice. A longer adjustment time might give the office opportunity to reinforce the value of its practice and successfully market that value to existing patients. Leadership skills will be needed in mature practices to not only manage the team but also the adjustment of the patients to the new dentist and the transition. Professionals who specialize in dental practice transitions need experience in developing the psychological factors necessary in retiring dentists to ensure successful transfer.

Gain Leadership Skills

How could you gain these skills? Many practice management companies provide online lectures. Network by attending a dental convention where this topic will be discussed and have conversations with convention exhibitors who specialize in transitions. Listen for tips to increase success, such as using precise communication, individual accountability, and impeccable execution and leadership. Additional skills such as poise, ingenuity, and ability to handle stressful situations always work well in a dental office, especially during transitions.

Transitions involve much more than economic and legal transfer of the practice. Successful change indicates the degree of interpersonal skills and professionalism of the whole team. Ideally, older dentists and hygienists will retire to teach these skills at universities, volunteer as board examiners, mentor, and provide leadership to graduating dentists and dental hygienists.

Start on a Job Course That Yields High Returns

As a new graduate, starting on a course that yields the greatest return in the least amount of time is far more effective than trying to figure it out as you go along. Clearly, the way people find jobs has changed in the past decades. Internet websites and dental employment agencies offer descriptions of employment opportunities. Some websites even require personality-type assessments.

If you walk into an office to give the dentist your résumé, call first and set up an appointment. Usually they will say they're not hiring, but dress for a business interview anyway. Attach a photo of yourself to the résumé. You want to set yourself apart as a person with a friendly smile. Express a desire to be considered for employment when someone is on sick leave or vacation if an opening for regular employment isn't available.

Networking with hygienists and dentists is vital to your success. After all, people do business with people they know, like, and trust. So exhibit a strong entrepreneurial spirit and explain your vision for how you want to practice. Develop a plan that the dentist and other dental hygienists will appreciate and recognize to be of worth. Ask to join a study club to showcase clinical skills, develop positive relationships, or share ideas to create a scheduling system that makes sense and makes a profit. The dentist wants to make sure you can keep a full schedule before you are hired.

What tools of technology do other hygienists use to keep the appointment schedule full? Knowing what resources are available when you go for an interview allows you to market yourself effectively and develop a relationship with the dentist. Doing this indicates you are "teachable" and can solve problems when given the opportunity.

Negotiate for More Money After You've Been Hired

In this example, the hygienist, a new graduate, is paid a starting rate of $31.25 an hour. The dentist's production rate can be calculated at $712,500 minus $180,000, which is a difference of $532,500. If the difference were divided by the 220 days that the office is open, for example, then the dentist's goal would be $2,420 daily.

The dentist originally wanted a $150,000 yearly hygiene production. Because the hygienist has had $15,000 higher production for six months ($2,500 additional production per month), negotiating with the dentist for a higher payment is reasonable.

With that amount of additional profit, numerous calculations can be used to figure what belongs to the hygienist, but communication has to start at some point. If the hygiene department's schedule is full and the dentist's schedule is not, this results in lower total daily production goals for the office. The hygienist should have in writing or in a contract what percentage of profit should be returned in bonus money if production increases above the previous negotiated rate.

If that rate is sustainable (and has been for six months), this situation needs to be addressed. In the stated case, at the end of the year, the hygienist would have overproduced $30,000. Hygienists consider that any equipment or uniforms needed to perform their duties are to be paid by the dentist with their initial contracted salary, so this money is considered profit over and above the initial agreement.

What percentage of this money belongs to the hygienist? Well, here's where the negotiation begins.

The dentist will probably want the negotiations to stay in the 33 to 35 percent range, but nothing precludes the hygienist from asking for a higher percentage. A portion of this amount, approximately $5,000, can be contributed to the hygienist's personal retirement plan. Assuming the dentist will take two-thirds of the hygienist's earnings and spend it however he or she decides, this is an excellent time to negotiate new equipment and instruments.

Plan Your Own Retirement Fund

As a hygienist, you can contact an investment firm, set up an account, and start contributing to your own retirement plan yearly. If the dentist has a retirement plan for employees, the dental hygienist must be included in that plan under federal laws for 401(k) plans, so negotiate before you're employed and understand the office plan.

Goodwill results when profits by the hygiene department contribute to the retirement plan for all employees. This generates a positive work environment toward the hygiene department from all who work in the office. The assistants will come to understand that the hygiene department not only provides long-term benefits for the patients but long-term retirement benefits for the team. This practice strategy motivates those in the hygiene department to have a full schedule.

Take time to ask about and understand the dentist's pension plan. Some plans require you to be employed a number of years (up to four) before you're entitled to money set aside for employee benefits. If you're terminated before that time, the money reverts to the dentist or owner of the plan. The point is this: Don't depend solely on the dentist's plan for retirement. Having your own plan is wise.

The remainder of the money can be used to supplement monthly income, negotiate repayment of school loans, or even provide additional education. Let's say you are the hygienist in the previous example. To supplement your hourly rate, you'd divide the remaining $10,000 by the hours worked per year. For example, if you worked 1,600 hours per year, you would calculate a $6.25 hourly increase. Remember, this is money you made, and nothing precludes you from asking the dentist to contribute more than a $6.25 hourly raise. The $31.25 starting hourly wage plus a new negotiated raise of $7.75 agreed to by the dentist would result in a $39 hourly wage. You never know how much you're worth if you don't risk asking the dentist for a raise when the money comes from the dentist's percentage of profit. Do your research, present your figures, and keep it simple to calculate.

Calculate Financials Before You Say Yes

As noted earlier, get informed about the business end of the practice. Realize that hygiene production comprises 20 to 25 percent of the total production in a typical general practice, so a higher hygiene percentage offers more value to the practice. This percentage can be increased to 30 percent or more in practices aggressively using soft-tissue management procedures.

However, in times of transition, these procedures add inflated value to a practice, especially if the dentist is under-producing or slowing down before retirement. The economic downturn caused many dental practices to diminish in value. Remember, buyers care about the future earnings of a practice, not its past earnings. Therefore, the hygiene department in effect becomes a forecaster of future earnings. Hygiene procedures, especially in periodontal treatment, can be manipulated. When the new buyer of the dental office assumes the role of new dentist, only then does one experience representative figures. Hygiene is a department all to itself and is expected to produce earnings reflecting constant growth.

The key to a successful transition is a comprehensive, accurate practice appraisal. That requires you to build your successful transition on a foundation of facts, not guesses. Then your new owner will consider you trustworthy.

After Accepting the Job

When you're first hired, it's important to know the previous hygienist's production goal figures. Always ask to see production goals, especially if you'll be the only hygienist in the office. Note: Most dentists expect a production of three times the daily salary. For example, the dentist would like to hire at the rate of his previous hygienist, who produced $150,000 per year. The average range of production for a hygienist is between $150,000 and $200,000 per year. The dentist will pay $250 per day but would like $750 of collected production per day, or $150,000 a year of production. This salary represents $31.25 per hour.

Keep a recorded figure of daily production on your personal calendar or printed schedule. Every month, calculate your actual production and compare it to the production goal. After six months of employment, determine the total production of the office and multiply it by the percentage of uncollected amount. For example, if six months of production for the office is $400,000 and the uncollected amount was $20,000, then the office's net production must be reduced by 5 percent, which brings it to $380,000.

Know that net total production minus fixed costs equal profit. What does it cost to run an office? Let's say rent is $7,000 per month, or a yearly total of $84,000; salaries for four employees are estimated at $156,750; supplies, insurance, utilities, and pension plans are $152,000. From this, you can determine if the office is making enough profit for you to ask for a raise. Note: A good rule is that overhead costs should be about 65 percent of net production.

Granted, you may not have access to some of this information. However, when discussing raises and benefits such as number of earned days of vacation, sick time, and medical insurance, it can help if you have a record of what you produce and lost chair time.

Define Achievable Production

Determine if the hygiene department is producing the goals set by the dentist and dental hygienist (you). Each provider of care has a separate goal. For example, suppose the hygiene department over the last six months of employment has produced $90,000, and this figure is $15,000 higher than previously determined. If this production rate can be accomplished for another month and expenses remain stable, then a raise is in order.

Document realistic goals every day and communicate your goals on a monthly basis. Be transparent and ask for help when necessary to develop your skills. Seasoned dentists need to make allowances for dental hygienists and dental graduates who aren't yet able to work as rapidly as someone with years of experience.

Mentoring enhances the skills taught in dental and dental hygiene schools and develops the relationship between the dentist and the dental hygienist. The fact that you are making progress and achieving goals shows your genuine contribution. A positive outlook and open communication generate solutions and achievement. Thank your patients for allowing you to be their dental hygienist during this period of adjustment.

Business Within a Business

Consider the hygiene department to be a business within a business. You can lead by example in these ways:

- Define your vision and share it with your coworkers.

- Work with excellent advisors and mentors.

- Create a yearly business plan that defines your goals and budget.

- Be a part of morning team and department meetings with the dentist.

- Understand each employee's strengths and motivators.

- Hold employees accountable for appropriate behavior and job performance.

- Monitor practice vital signs monthly and expenses quarterly.

- Provide coaching to aid in success of the goals.

- Praise, appreciate, and recognize your colleagues and other employees regularly.

- Hold performance reviews quarterly on yourself (even if the dentist or owner doesn't).

Performance Goals

Performance goals are ones that make you reach just past your fingertips, but they're still achievable. Performance goals usually include numerical targets, making their achievement measureable. Learning goals can be educational, such as speaking a foreign language so you can communicate with patients, or learning how to sharpen instruments.

When you confuse performance and learning goals, you compromise your values and fail. For example, the dentist wants you to sharpen 10 instruments a day, but you don't know how to sharpen instruments so you learn the procedure first, then assign a numbers goal to practice.

A performance goal for the dental hygienist might be associated with the amount of revenue the dentist would like to generate. Perhaps the dentist would like to repeat a gross production of one million dollars in the next year, but to achieve this collective goal calls for deducting bad debt and making insurance adjustments.

Assuming production adjustments were five percent for the previous year, consider the following formulation: Divide the collection goal by the percentage of inverted adjustment. Therefore, the gross production goal of $1,000,000 divided by 95% = $1,052,632. The new monthly goal for the next year is $1,052,632 divided by 12 = $87,719 monthly.

Each provider of care has a separate goal. The hygiene salary is based on a daily salary of $250, and the dentist would like production to be three times salary so the hygienist needs to produce $750 per day. If the hygienist works 220 days a year, the hygienist would produce $165,000 toward the total production goal of a million dollars. If the office has two hygienists, the production would be doubled to $330,000 for the total hygiene department. The dentist's part would be $670,000, or the difference. Divide the difference by the 220 days the dentist will work, and the dentist's daily goal would be $3,045.

Performance goals are a team effort, and each person's performance counts. Breaking down performance goals with the dentist can indicate whether the ideas are realistic. You want achievable results that empower the team.

The hygiene department needs accurate record keeping, including independent records, separate from the dental software. These records are handy to have for performance reviews. Keep records of your total production figures monthly. Work with the administrative person at the front desk to separate by procedure the hygienist's portion of the charges. Give credit for only what the hygienist performs, and this does not include exams. It does include radiographs, whitening, periodontal treatments, and fluoride treatments. Know the codes of the procedures you perform and the charges for those codes.

Every three months, calculate the amount of lost revenue. For example, if you have 1,250 active patients multiplied by two (two appointments each a year), then to make this goal, you need 2,500 appointments a year. Say each hygienist had 1,760 appointments (multiplied by two, that's 3,520 appointments). That means the hygiene department potentially lost 1,020 appointments (3,520 minus 2,500). Then multiply 1,020 by the average fee (say $100) to equal $102,000. This amount represents the lost revenue for the practice in a year.

Every hour of lost production is vital to the office overhead. In this example, each hygienist would have had 510 appointments a year (about two a day) that went unfilled. This is why so many dentists require the dental hygienist to see 10 patients a day. The dentist can't subsidize the hygiene department or hire another hygienist unless the demand for work is well documented.

If you have more than one unfilled hour of production time a day, this figure represents an area for improvement. Consider these questions:

- Do you have the help of the team to fill lost production time?

- Was the patient reminded well in advance of the appointment?

- Would fees associated with a service that reminds patients of appointments be worth the investment?

- Who or what are the causes for lost appointments?

- Are office hours incompatible with patients' work hours?

- Does the office need appointments on Saturday?

- What are the reasons given by the patients for not coming into the office for routine maintenance?

- Does the patient understand why the appointment with the hygienist is critical to the overall health of the patient?

- Has the patient had other broken appointments in the office?

Continue to ask questions of the dentist and team members until the solution is uncovered to make sure every hour is productive.

Additionally, every three months, calculate the number of days of production needed and see if this figure is diminishing or increasing. How can you sell yourself to the dentist and team if you don't know what the future scheduling needs are for the office? You'll also need an active patient scheduling report. Active patients are patients who have been in the office for hygiene appointments in the last year.

The following example indicates 20 percent will be lost to normal patient attrition. How many three-, four-, six-month recall appointments will be needed in the future?

The office has a total of 1000 returning patients, and they're separated into the following categories:

- Three-month recall: 20 patients x 4 times a year = 80 appointments

- Four-month recall: 30 patients x 3 times a year = 90 appointments

- Six-month recall: 900 patients x 2 times a year = 1,800 appointments

- One year recall: 50 patients x 1 time a year = 50 appointments

= 2,020 appointments

Now estimate half of last year's number of new patient appointments. For example, 10 patients a month times 12 months equals 120. Therefore, you'll need to add 60 appointments to the estimate, which generates 2,080 appointments. This number divided by 220 days (or the number of days you worked in a year) equals 9.45 patients each day. That means the hygienist is encouraged to see more patients than eight a day. With this example, the dentist might think that a second hygienist is unnecessary, especially if the retention rate cannot be stabilized.

Periodontal therapy courses could increase knowledge of why some patients need to be on three- and four-month recall. From this example of 2,080 appointments, a four-day work week is still necessary. Estimates indicate that the production will now equal that of last year despite attrition; however, the hygiene department may want to strive for at least a five percent growth rate each year in order to add additional personal.

Stay connected to your patient. Use patient engagement technologies and software programs that integrate texting to help you retain, reactivate, and acquire patients. Be persistent and detailed with your records because an active base can take up to five years to develop. Keeping records is vital to growth and achieving raises.

Retention Rate

Another consideration of the hygiene department is the retention rate of the practice. Do more patients leave out the back door than come in through the front door?

Hygienists are instrumental to the practice because people want stability. It's more difficult to attract new patients than it is to retain an existing patient. Let's say you had 120 new patients for the year but only 60 came back for six-month recall, which means you had a 50 percent retention rate. For every two people who came through the front door, one left out the back door. This is not acceptable. This rating is shared by the whole office team, so each member should be aware and try and improve the rating to the 80-90 percent retention level.

Calculate retention rate as the actual number of recall patients treated divided by the recall patients due. In this case, if 1,800 six-month recall patients were treated but 2,080 recall patients were due, then 1,800 divided by 2,080 is 86 percent. Remember, retention is the basis for good solid growth every year, and you want to grow the practice by 7-10 percent each year. These are examples of performance goals. Now what is a learning goal?

Learning Goals

A dentist with whom I was employed suggested that a dental assistant be in the room with the patient during a consultation appointment. How would the office achieve this new requirement? A dental assistant would take consultation notes, monitor blood pressure, and attend to communication with the patient and the dentist. Would we need to hire someone to be with the dentist and patient, or did we need to look at individual work steps of the team?

We studied what was happening before the patient was brought into the room for consultation. This dentist had a team of four employees—two receptionists and two assistants. Where were the team members when the dentist was giving a consultation? The whole team assessed the problem, discussed the problem, and came up with an experiment that worked. The key to the solution? All members were engaged.

This kind of problem solving and learning makes teams happy and maintains interest in the job. Team members are the masters of their own fate and they develop self-efficacy. No office manager was needed to dictate the event. No politics were involved and no harsh communication. The conversation involved: "Do you think this should be a priority that will make this office more efficient and productive? Let's work together to come up with suggestions. I know if we brainstorm, we can solve this issue." This is an example of a team learning goal. In this case, we redirected one receptionist to be with the doctor. New technology that involved purchasing a tablet computer was learned and the information was directly submitted into a treatment plan, which reduced errors. It was a win-win solution for everyone involved.

Questions to Consider

- What American Dental Association procedures can you complete? What are the codes and dollar amounts for these procedures?

- Do you know the definitions of the procedure codes so you can accurately code procedures for submission to insurance?

- How often do you review your production figures with your dentist to ensure accuracy?

- Why are production, active-patient figures, and retention rates important?

- When did you last review the market to identify patient engagement technologies that remind patients of appointments or other technological advancements?

- When did you last set production goals for yourself?

- When did you last set learning goals for yourself?

- When did your office last set a learning goal for the team?

- If your hygiene department is growing, what accounting can you provide to validate the need to employ additional hygienists?

- How active are you in growing the hygiene department in times of decline?

- What is the budget set by the dentist in your office for improvements made to the hygiene department?

Negotiating a Raise After You've Landed the Job

From the previous production figures stated and a yearly estimated profit in the hygiene department of $30,000, I suggest you start negotiation above $6.75 per hour because below that rate is not a raise. Of that profit, how much can go to a sustainable raise? If there is agreement on $10,000, then that figure divided by 220 days worked is $45.00 of added salary per day. Now divide $295 by 8 and you have an average of $37.00 per hour. The new hourly salary is therefore $31.25 plus $6.75, which equals $37.00 per hour. How much is the dentist willing to contribute? This is where the real negotiation starts. The dentist might say "seven" and you might say "nine," so you agree on an eight-dollar raise per hour, realizing the dentist would like to see if the process can be repeated. Accurate record keeping and documentation are important. If you can, renegotiate in three months and again at the end of the year. In this case, you are contributing at a higher percentage of three times your salary, which generates more profit for the dentist.

This example indicates that if a yearly salary for the dental hygienist started at $50,000, through proper financial data, the salary could be increased to between $60,000 and $65,000 depending on the negotiated hourly increase and number of days employed. With production of $180,000 minus an uncollected amount, the dental hygienist is more than paying for the expenses of supplies and rent of the office. But don't assume the dentist will accept your figures. Make sure you're both in agreement of how a fair salary is earned and taxes are paid.

Most hygienists continue to work for a straight 33 to 35 percent of hygiene production. This is a perfectly acceptable way of earning salary as long as taxes, vacation, sick leave, and other benefits are accumulated every payday.

Suppose you developed the baseline as a new hygienist and now have moved up to a more experienced level. Knowing how to base your salary on production and negotiate raises is important in achieving remuneration based on what you're worth to the practice. This type of communication develops a colleague relationship with the dentist.

If the level of production is achievable and consistent in the previous example, then the hygiene department is growing by a yearly rate of 20 percent. After the raise, it would be appropriate for the dentist to consider hiring a second hygienist on a part-time basis to handle the excessive growth. Ultimately, you want to keep the balance of the office engaged in a full schedule, while connecting with patients and becoming comfortable with the process of delivering care.

Approximately 40 percent of dentists do not employ a hygienist. It's a shame because patients who are afraid to see the dentist benefit from receiving care from another professional who should be able to make them feel comfortable. Perhaps more participation and acknowledgment of the business goals for the practice will increase the growth of hygiene opportunities. Simply indicating you are aware of the risk provides an opportunity (in most cases) to sell yourself to a dentist who will take a chance and hire you.

Develop Solid Financial Habits

It's wise to scrutinize the details of your personal finances as well as your professional finances. Often, successful professionals can recall in extreme detail every dollar spent and all revenue earned at their job; however, ask them how much they allocate for housing, transportation, personal spending, and savings, and they have no clue. They often don't even know how much debt they owe. Budgets provide accountability. According to the American Dental Association's 2010 Survey on Investments and Retirement, the average dentist saves about $26,000 per year, 17 percent of net income, and realizes it's not enough. Most dentists and dental hygienists want to make more money to meet expenses, but the best predict-tor of financial security is how much you know about and control your budget.

A simple rule for budget division is: 35 percent for housing, 15 percent for transportation, 25 percent for personal expenditures, 15 percent to pay off debt, and 10 percent for savings. If you budget your time during a patient appointment, it only makes sense to budget your money in the office as well as your personal expenses. When dentist and hygienist mirror budget efforts in the office, results can produce significant opportunities to improve the practice and secure maximum profit.

When your earnings go up, then increase your savings and retirement plans. Watch out, though. You can have too much confidence that things will go as planned. You can never be absolutely positive your health will never deteriorate, your business will never lose value, the stock market will always go up, or real estate will never lose value. Many people have learned that the hard way. It's best to protect yourself for retirement (or your next endeavor) by establishing good financial habits early on. Allow those plans to be flexible to adapt to an unforeseen future.

Contribute to a retirement plan the first day you start work. Find an investment firm that will help you define your goals and then make consistent contributions. Determining a retirement age in advance will help you achieve your goals. If you know what you should be paid based on what you're capable of producing, you can maximize your financial situation.

Be Prepared for Transitions

Once you've gained employment, you'll want to keep it in times of transition, so remain aware of business details. When a dentist sells the practice, it's important to have updated dental hygiene practice information. Accurate records indicating charges, payments, adjustments, and the profits of the hygiene department for at least the past three years are required. Many other items of information are also necessary when the possibility of hiring a new associate dentist arises or the dentist wants to sell and retire. These include: a written statement of practice philosophy; copies of the policy and procedures manuals and OSHA records manual; a description of marketing used to attract patients; and information on the geographic area where the practice is located.

Even if your dentist has the best of intentions, derailment can occur as a result of family illness or a change in health or marital status. The best course of action is to be aware of the business climate so in times of uncertainty you can continue your employment in which you've invested time. Listen and ask questions when you have discussions with the dentist or when financial and production information is shared.

The business policies of corporate dentistry, or even dentists who own more than two dental offices, have changed the scope of private practice for dentists. Private practices survive on the goodwill and referrals of their patients. It's the relationship forged by the team that gains the practice's long-term reputation and people's trust. No one can be in two places at the same time; ownership is necessary. A young dentist staying for two to three years at a practice and leaving for a better financial opportunity doesn't provide long-term growth. When practices emphasize quantity of patients rather than quality of time spent with them, an exponential decline may occur in patient satisfaction. Sometimes spending an extra 30 minutes with a patient to explain existing problems is worth more to the practice than performing an exam on a new patient.

Consistent growth as measured by annual revenue indicates the strength of the practice. A good benchmark for growth is 7 to 10 percent growth annually. This can even be higher with an effective marketing plan in operation. A new graduate has no experience in retaining existing patients, reactivating lost patients, and acquiring new patients, whereas an experienced hygienist can be instrumental in building the growth of the practice. Patients feel quite comfortable visiting a dental office where the dental hygienist is familiar, approachable, caring, and obviously experienced.

Thus, developing communication and business skills can help provide guidance and success for the practice you're in as well as ensure your employment.

Further Issues That May Arise

To forecast how you might practice in the future, look at the following trends. The North Texas area is fortunate to have Baylor College of Dentistry. Suggestions on how to practice can be based on the statistics and the many articles on the future evolution of dental teams by Dr. Eric Solomon, mentioned previously. In his 2004 article on dental economics, Dr. Solomon cites statistics that suggest the dental hygiene profession will experience massive expansion of up to 44 percent. Therefore, it seems future dental hygienists will need to be quite inventive with issues of employment. Increased numbers of dental hygienists could make long-term employment difficult; therefore budgets and retirement planning become essential.

Might the ethics of dental hygiene be tested because of an inability to withstand the effects of disruptions in employment? One can always find a critic who says newly graduated dentists and dental hygienists can't produce enough to make expenses. They're said to be too "teacher-like" to make it as a clinician, or too introverted, or too selfish, and the list goes on. Hostile comments and excessive demands on professionals for productivity make for poor work environments. Diminishing the strength of dental hygienists by encouraging fraud or selling unnecessary products and procedures will erode public trust. No such environment should be allowed to compromise ethics. However, at some point when a job is needed, a hygienist could be tempted to take any job and deal with ethics and environment later.

Aim for a Stable Environment

Never before in the history of dental hygiene education has it been more important to teach and understand how to create a stable environment. The 2009 recession caused massive job losses and dental hygienists' hours were drastically reduced as dentists adjusted to the transition. Active engagement is not an easy concept to communicate, but it's about being the protector of a stable environment in times of crisis, which becomes necessary to keep the practice viable.

In case of the death or prolonged illness of your lead dentist, for example, it's wise to develop an action plan based on communication that can be trusted, but know your boundaries. Other common causes for absences are disability due to accident, surgery, pregnancy, substance abuse, illness, and death of a spouse or family member. Retaining knowledgeable experts even when the dentist will be returning requires planning to ensure financial security. Practice disruptions longer than two weeks without a dentist can call for decisive action for a temporary associate to aid the list of emergency dentists. Local employment agencies, practice brokers, and consultants can be sources of help to the hygienist and family.

I encourage you to be a level-headed leader in times of crisis and work closely with the dentist's family. Organize other practitioners who will aid the office as temporary emergency dentists. If necessary, secure a broker who can help the dentist's family transition the office to an associate dentist who can assume leadership. Planning for a crisis is one of the most thoughtful actions you can take to help family and team members survive in a period of grief. The practice depends on a hygienist who can develop a "story line" that's been approved by the family and broker. That means communicating effectively in a business-as-usual attitude by keeping the same hours and team members.

Let me stress again that it's critical to maintain the stability of the practice, whether the owner will be returning from a prolonged illness or another dentist will buy the practice. Most dental offices have passwords for the top administrator level of practice software. Encourage the dentist to also have someone outside of the office in possession of the password, such as the accountant and family members. Every online business account has a password, so if you are trusted with this information, chances are the dentist would also consider you to be trusted with the action plan in times of disruption. Issues such as grief in case of death involve retaining knowledgeable experts who can make realistic decisions for the future of the practice. Advisors may include an accountant, banker, financial advisor, and attorney, as well as key consultants such as a broker who can offer realistic options to the family for the practice. Preserving the practice preserves the memories and the security of the team, and also helps with the grieving process. Engage advisors so that you can make a goal to provide for your secure future.

Keep Looking Forward

Do you remember how much you wanted the job? You thanked the dentist for the interview and ended with your many qualifications deemed important to the success of the business.

Now that you have the job, be sure to set realistic production and learning goals, strive to stay ahead of the business changes, improve your clinical skills, and keep engaged with technology. Setting and achieving your goals will give you satisfaction as you see the progress you're making. Your work can be a significant factor in the success of the practice.

CHAPTER 4: EDUCATING HYGIENISTS TODAY

"The beautiful thing about learning is that no one can take it away from you."

– B.B. King

Associate dental hygiene degree programs provide the same basic training as Bachelor of Science degree programs because all must be accredited by the American Dental Association (ADA) and meet ADA standards. Associate degree and bachelor degree programs are required by the Commission on Dental Accreditation (CODA) to include a minimum number of clinical hours. The major differences between these programs are in the public health, research, and general education courses. Bachelor of Science programs require more hours of general education, including exposure to history, literature, and the arts. Additional education by baccalaureate programs can provide the hygienist with business and problem-solving skills as well as life-long learning. The regional and state licensure boards test the basic entry-level skills and knowledge of hygienists. Associate degree hygienists should strive to also obtain a bachelor's of science degree to ensure progression in their career. The proliferation of schools may lead to an over-supply of hygienists. Therefore, skills, additional education, and ethical behavior become even more important.

The American Dental Hygiene Association (ADHA) has three categories of membership: active, retired and allied. Retired status has an age requirement of 65 years. However, the ADHA doesn't recognize the past education and license of a dental hygienist who has retired her clinical license before the age of 65 as being active and now retired status. This makes a difference if the retired hygienist's desire is to serve on a board or mentor students at a school. Not every hygienist is clinical, as options for employment include sales, office management, and consulting. I suggest the ADHA dismiss the age requirement and recognize hygienists as having retired status if their license has been retired. I'd like to see the ADHA be active in changing bylaws to provide an accurate representation of the organization. This association could allow hygienists employed in other areas of dentistry such as practice management or sales to serve as delegates and be active in their local organizations.

Dental and dental hygiene schools are reluctant to allow retired professionals who aren't members of the ADHA to mentor or coach students. I see this wealth of knowledge being wasted. Schools often require membership because accreditation requires a professional component, which is easier to obtain if faculty or mentors are members of the ADHA. In fact, schools get awards based on the percentage of faculty membership. If our profession is to provide jobs, let's not waste expanded education after dental or dental hygiene school; this expansion is necessary for the survival of the profession.

The medical industry has embraced the concept of expansion in education with the addition of the nurse practitioner and the physician assistant. Nursing is moving forward to require all entry-level licensure to include a bachelor's of science (BS) degree. Pharmacy, physical therapy, and occupational therapy will soon require a doctoral degree for their entry-level education credentials.

The trend in dentistry is for more Bachelor of Science dental hygiene programs to close and more associate programs to open. I believe this decision is moving the profession of dental hygiene in the wrong direction. Master of Science degree programs in dental hygiene emphasizing tracks in business management and independent practice are needed. Starting doctoral dental hygiene pro-grams in a dental school would provide a setting to train hygienists to conduct research relative to gingivitis and periodontitis.

Periodontal disease has been associated with systemic diseases such as heart disease, respiratory disease, and diabetes. New tech-nologies that provide minimally invasive, nonsurgical treatment in periodontics could be offered by hygienists. Nothing is gained by diluting education—certainly not better dental care—and nothing is gained in education if standards aren't enforced and improved.

Pros and Cons of a Hygienist-Focused Practice

Some dentists would like legally office-trained dental assistants to do many of the procedures that only hygienists are allowed to do, such as scaling and polishing of supramarginal tooth surfaces. Supporting the lowest possible level of education for dental hygienists might be attractive to dentists because salaries in private practice are tied in large part to services provided. Dentists certainly won't support independent dental hygiene private practice if they see it as business competition. Hygienists in these independent practices would probably have higher educational degrees and be specifically trained in their skill area. Employment of dental hygienists in schools, nursing homes, hospitals, and university research could expand opportunities for dentists. Irrespective of public health or private practice, dentists rely on the skills of dental hygienists to diagnose restorative care and those off-site patients could be re-ferred to a dentist who would continue restorative treatment. Many states—Michigan, Minnesota, Washington, Colorado, and New Mexico—provide dental hygienists opportunities to work in public health with minimal supervision. Legalizing independent practices for hygienists in all states with additional education pro-grams and credentialing by a state board would greatly expand opportunities for growth of the overall industry.

The Texas Oral Health Coalition (TxOHC) was formed in 2004 to address oral health issues across the state and ensure that every citizen enjoys optimum oral health. The Coalition is composed of medical and dental professionals, community agencies, faith-based organizations, policy developers, insurance companies, professional educators, and state and other governmental entities. Dentists and dental hygienists share a common goal of improving oral healthcare. With a mission to actively promote collaborative efforts, neither the Texas Dental Association (TDA) nor the Texas Dental Hygienists' Association (TDHA) has any special status. This helps alleviate any possible interpretation that either group of professionals has more influence on the coalition than the other.

What Effects Do the ADA, ADHA, and AGD have on Your Practice?

Over the years, the American Dental Association (ADA) has established rigorous testing guidelines for dental products, including toothpastes, mouthwashes, toothbrushes, and other products for dental use. Manufacturers voluntarily submit their products to the ADA for testing so their products can join the more than 1,300 products that proudly display the Seal of Acceptance. The ADA works to educate the public about oral health through patient education pamphlets, websites, and public service announcements. It established National Children's Health Month in an effort to promote dental health for kids.

The Academy of General Dentistry (AGD) is a dental organization created on February 6, 1952, by general dentists who met in Chicago to create and sign what would be the first charter. These dentists identified a vacancy in the dental profession: No established, consolidated source existed to provide dentists with continuing education (CE) opportunities. Since then, the academy has grown to become the second-largest dental association in the

U.S., behind the ADA, with a mission to advance the value and excellence of general dentistry.

Membership in the American Dental Hygiene Association (ADHA) may influence hygienists through exposure to current research in disease transmission. Education is vital to effect change in the attitudes and practices of dental hygienists when treating patients with infectious or "unknown" diseases. Greater access to research publications and continuing education programs through local, state, and national associations may make members more knowledgeable about infectious disease transmission, decreasing contamination and increasing the trust of the public by altering clinical practices to adhere to strict sterilization guidelines. Hygienists are exposed to research that compares pre- and post-access to dental care for low-income, underserved, or unserved populations, and this research is vital should legislation be passed that affects the dental industry.

Whenever I have questions about my profession, I survey members of the ADA, AGD, or ADHA for current analysis and alliance. These organizations provide insight on how dentists and dental hygienists work and think about problems by providing research articles and viewpoints. Why do I suggest becoming a ADHA member? Because the ADHA represents advances in clinical communication, mutual cooperation, and representation that serves professional interests across the country. From water fluoridation to the dental accreditation programs, the ADA, AGD, and ADHA are involved in everything related to dentistry.

About 70 percent of dentists in the U.S. belong to the ADA. Since 1859, the organization has developed standards for the educational requirement of dentists and the accreditation of dental and dental hygiene schools. It has funded dental research, increased dental coverage from Medicaid and Children's Health Insurance Programs (CHIP), and reduced dental costs through insurance reforms. Approximately 150,000 members contribute yearly dues of $500 with nine percent of total dues going to lobbying efforts. Every specialty has its own organization, but for over 60 years, the Academy of General Dentists (AGD) has tracked the continuing education units (CEUs) members earn to help them meet their state licensure requirements and represents about 30 percent membership. Membership in the ADHA is below 50 percent of hygienists. Continued decreases in membership will create a questionably viable future path for the organizations, one that will for sure affect leadership.

Headquarters for all these organizations are seven minutes from each other in Chicago, but philosophies of the AGD and ADHA can be overshadowed by the ADA, which has $137 million in assets. If the ADA forged alliances with the AGD and ADHA, it could reduce fees and overhead while focusing on long-term planning, which is much overdue. Organizations must work together to improve relationships, but that has not been the case in dentistry. Sharing power in the medical model starts from earliest training in hospitals, where tasks are delegated among nurses, physician assistants, phlebotomists, and radiologists. This kind of culture doesn't exist in dentistry, but it could if members decide they want it.

Organizations working together would redefine the culture of dentistry. In the dental office, the dentist and the dental hygienist work together to meet the oral health needs of patients. Each state has its own specific regulations regarding the hygienist's responsibility. Gender in dental schools is fairly evenly balanced with an equal percentage of male and female dental applicants. In contrast, dental hygiene schools are 95 percent female. It's hoped that more males will see a future as dental hygienists, as they have in the nursing profession. Male dental hygienists are especially needed in Veterans Administration (VA) hospitals and military bases.

When there's an economic downturn, dentists and hygienists displaced from employment wonder if payment of ADA and ADHA dues are justified given the services rendered. When faced with a limited budget, professionals start to ask "What are these organizations doing for me?"

Active participation in dental and dental hygiene organizations is the best way to keep up with clinical, ethical, and leadership skills. The Texas Practice Act was amended a few years ago to require a set number of hours of continuing education units, or CEUs, for license renewal. The ADHA offers an abundance of online courses for which continuing education units can be attained. If you find a lack of course materials you're interested in, then develop them and submit articles to the ADHA. Noninvasive periodontal therapy will utilize periodontist and dental hygienist team concepts, and the American Academy of Periodontology (AAP) offers a yearly Dental Hygiene Symposium. Many of the abstracts are available for viewing on the website; take time to learn from them.

As mentioned earlier, almost no business or leadership courses are taught in dental, dental hygiene, or dental assisting schools. After graduation, faced with managing their own practice, many dentists and dental hygienists rely on practice managers or dental supply equipment companies for knowledge. This needs to change. With organizations already providing the required CEU clinical courses, non-clinical business courses need to be added to develop the necessary leadership skills to retain a license.

The effectiveness of the leadership of a dentist or dental hygienist can be measured through general patient satisfaction and through feedback from the people they supervise. Effectiveness includes the ability to share information, be involved in decision making, coach, provide feedback, mediate conflicts, be trustworthy, and be confident in one's clinical abilities. These skills and qualities must be reinforced constantly every year.

Certainly, changes in technology take time to develop, learn, and implement. Perceptions and behaviors change daily as we are bombarded with decisions. We may not even realize we are vulnerable to changing ethics and compromise.

With Collaboration, Our Influence Spreads

Freud, Einstein, and Churchill changed the world. They developed or led huge numbers of people to reach new understandings through their insights. They challenged thinking in new and different ways. The world would be different without the influence of these men.

We, too, can have influence in our own segment of the world and industry. What could we learn from one another if each dentist or dental hygienist made a goal to submit one article for publication to educate others? As a result, the promotion of optimal oral health might have more preventive focus. Teamwork and collaboration between dentist and dental hygienist might also be restored or enhanced.

Professional organizations can promote the dentist, hygienist, assistant, and any support team member working together to realize shared goals. One way to do this is to offer awards. For example, research and publications written by a dentist and dental hygienist would allow for joint intellectual problem solving. A publication written by a dentist, office team member, and a dental laboratory employee or researcher might offer tips on improving crown restorations.

The American Academy of Periodontology (AAP) was formed in 1914 by two women. What other women have made great advances in dentistry? Women in dental history or children's dental care might be topics for book awards sponsored through the various dental organizations.

Writing a book preserves the profession, and ideas could be infinitely generated with the support of these professional organizations. Collaboration by promoting ways to exchange ideas and research should always be a top priority of the ADA.

However, as organizations grow in strength and power, they begin to lose sight of how dentistry is provided to the public. The organization grows and hires good people to run the business and provide member services. Pretty soon these people are preparing the agendas and sitting at the elbows of the elected dental members, "helping" them guide the organization in the "right" direction. Human greed can then overcome their interest in supporting the members. Staff members naturally want more dues, political power, bigger departments, and higher salaries. They begin to work for themselves instead of the members or the organization.

The ADA bylaws establish the mechanism for the Certified Dental Terminology (CDT) by establishing the Code Maintenance Committee (CMC), a body that includes representatives from other dental specialty organizations and third-party insurance providers. Therefore, the ADA charges fees for promoting and licensing coding products. CMC members vote to accept, amend, or decline CDT code-change requests. CDT code maintenance is warranted. However, offering awards to private practices and academia to jointly solve problems, have conversations, and motivate individual dentists or even dental hygienists to take action might better connect the ADA to its members. It's possible that leadership could emerge from all levels within and outside of the organization. However, when an individual expects to have a career with the ADA, it leaves little time to be directly involved with patient care, which influences many dentists to not belong to the organization. A mechanism for connecting private practice, public health, and professionals who are providing services every day is needed to reconnect members of the ADA.

Awards in dentistry similar to the Nobel Peace Prize but for innovative economic dental business models, procedures, technologies, and dental materials might spur collaborative efforts between dentists and dental laboratories or dental hygienists.

Monetary awards might provide a grant or secure employment in private practice and allow for growth in the industry.

Individuals aren't required to have a dental background to be employed by the ADA, but an organization should never lose sight of the members it represents and how those members go to work every day to supply dentistry to the public.

Professional organizations overlap, just as services provided by the dentist overlap those provided by the hygienist. Therefore, it is critical to learn how to exchange ideas. It might mean preserving the integrity of the industry.

When we represent an organization, it's of utmost importance to create alliances to promote understanding of problems in dentistry. The purpose of representation is not to protect our own specialty in dentistry. Learning is more cross-functional than ever before in hospitals. Physicians and surgical teams learn and practice together. Nurse practitioners partner with companies such as Johnson and Johnson for nursing hospice care. Foundations such as the W. K. Kellogg Foundation help support the Children's Dental Health Project in Washington, D.C. by providing grants for operating expenses. Companies need healthy employees and look to the dental industry as partners in keeping a healthy workforce.

If universities provide training and education for jobs in the field of dentistry, then dentists and dental hygienists need to become creative in how to provide care and employment opportunities. The dental industry needs continued initiation of grants to study specific areas of underutilization and clinical concerns. Research to improve dentistry and provide more employment opportunities are needed to spark creativity and forge more relationships. How will the ADA or ADHA know the concerns if there's no mechanism for debate and proposal?

You are part of that progress—the most important part—because, collectively, the organizations would not exist without shared respect and love for this industry.

Questions to Consider

- How do you view the importance of the hygienist in dentistry?

- What do you consider your own challenges moving forward and how can you address them?

- How do you see your role expanding?

- In what ways can you educate others on the role of dental hygiene?

CHAPTER 5: DEFINING PROFESSIONALISM IN DENTISTRY

"Be the change you want to see in the world."

– Gandhi

A dental hygienist is a preventive oral healthcare professional and a dentist is a restorative oral healthcare professional. Both professionals have completed an accredited program, passed a written national board examination, and successfully performed clinical skills on a state or regional examination. Professionals make it their business to know their business.

Application of new skills learned in dental or dental hygiene school can be overwhelming when you take those skills to the workplace. How do you select the right practice in which to be employed, and how do you become part of the dental team? Teachers surrounded you in school, but in your first job, you may experience a feeling of isolation. Have you been trained enough? Do you have the confidence to believe you can do it? Now is when the real education begins.

The Role of Ethics

Ethics determine how we practice. Ethics is how we agree to behave in a particular situation. Certain conduct is associated with professionalism and sets the bar for how we act and react. Training improves reaction time when the situation is an emergency.

For example, a Fort Worth, Texas, dental hygienist demonstrated professionalism when a car crashed into the dental office. Julie Watson rushed to the scene, where two men had pulled the driver out of the car and placed him on the grass in front of the office. Watson saw the driver was unconscious and had no pulse; his whitish-blue color indicated the diagnosis of a heart attack. She was totally in control and yelled for people to bring gloves, towels, and the clinic's automated external defibrillator. Shocking the man once with the defibrillator, she then started cardiopulmonary resuscitation (CPR) and felt relieved to see the color come back into his face. Emergency responders praised Watson's coolness and expertise. Her knowledge and skill had been gained as a dental hygienist trained in emergency procedures.

The challenge for professionalism is that most problems are complex. Daily, we are faced with multiple right choices, so what is the best right choice? If we make this choice, who and what does that choice affect? If we accept employment with Dr. A, how will the sterilization techniques be handled if our ethics and values are different? How will we be open to change if Dr. A expects our clinical skills to change from what we learned in school? Will we be willing to learn how to work differently with new challenges? How will our efforts affect the desire for increased production in the office? We can't answer these questions until we're faced with the situation.

Good interpersonal skills are critical in developing professionalism. However, additional components include knowledge, time management, appearance, communication skills, confidence, and personal ethics as well as a good work ethic. These are elements of professionalism relevant every day in every career.

Stories of Professionalism

Molly Whalen, a 2011 Forsyth School of Dental Hygiene graduate, began her reign as Miss Massachusetts 2011 at the 72nd Annual Miss Massachusetts Scholarship Pageant. During her year of service, she highlighted her platform, Smart Smiles: Promoting the Importance of Oral Health. She also promoted The Children's Miracle

Network Hospitals, the national platform of the Miss America organization. Molly fulfilled her responsibilities as Miss Massachusetts while she pursued a master's degree in applied nutrition at Northeastern University. She's an example of professionalism initially learned by obtaining a dental hygiene degree.

Stories of professionalism abound, such as those about dentists and dental hygienists who moved to Alaska to work for the Indian Health Service. Helping Alaskan natives obtain desperately needed dental care involve life-changing experiences and personal sacrifices.

Hurricane Katrina, in 2005, also brought out examples of professionalism. This hurricane caused one of the largest and most abrupt relocations of people in U.S. history. Many people came to Texas requiring emergency dental treatment. One of the many that touched me personally was a 12-year-old girl in pain because a molar tooth was decayed to the point she needed emergency treatment. Standing outside the treatment room, her parents decided an extraction was necessary after discussion with the dentist. But in the room, the little girl in the dental chair softly asked a dental hygienist if the tooth could be saved. She needed to have the options explained and trusted the person who touched her hand. After exploring the options, she signaled to others so she could express her wishes, and the treatment plan was altered and approved by her parents. A telephone call was made and the patient was referred for endodontic treatment.

In this case, professionals came together and made the best decision with the information presented and probability for success. However, grey areas exist in which treatment plans can go in different directions with health complexities beyond dental issues. Dentists and dental hygienists value treatment plans they formulate with patients. Many patients displaced by Hurricane Katrina needed medical surgeries. Hospitals and communities were challenged, but with time and awareness, Texas citizens provided results that were astonishing. Overcoming a daunting task and offering access to care in the face of a hurricane exhibits values of concern, stewardship, and justice. A professional gives options to others who suffer and teaches people how to prevent disease and live healthier lives, but the patient is the one who decides.

The Importance of Team Support

The dentists who employed me cared about learning and encouraged their hygienists to work collectively and achieve goals. They worked with me when I didn't know how to expand my thoughts or skills, continued to inspire me, and always asked, "What do you think about this?"

The best leaders implement step-by-step systems that help maximize the skills of each team member. They believe in you and you start to believe in yourself. The team members promote self-efficacy, the belief that you can do what you want to do with your life. They communicate that they care about your progress. The way to increase self-efficacy is to have a role model, learn how to deal with stress, and start to have mastery experiences by breaking down your goals into tiny goals that you can achieve.

Great dentists that broaden experiences allow hygienists to develop additional skills beyond dental hygiene. For me, practice management in an oral surgery office was my next career advancement. Diagnosis of the issue when a patient telephones an oral surgery office can be complicated, but my previous employer dentists provided exceptional training. Because I knew the symptoms and issues, many a dentist would lovingly call me "Dr. Deborah," and this viewpoint connected me with the patient and general dentist and expanded my body of work.

Role of Practice Manager

Moving from dental hygienist into the role of practice manager is an easy progression in the dental industry because experience has been gained in marketing a dental hygiene practice with both patient and dentist coordination. This knowledge base gives the hygienist an advantage as practice manager. Dentists know their patients they've referred to specialists for additional care are properly cared for when good communication exists between offices. Coordination of the case can involve hospitalization with an anesthesiologist or even multiple specialists. Hygienists in the role of practice managers understand the complex cases and the time constraints that affect communication. Dentists have ultimate responsibility for the practice, and provide the best dentistry they can, all of which can dictate the degree of communication. Dental hygienists in an office manager role have the training and experience to shoulder some of this responsibility. A professional who has good communication skills and knowledgeable of changes in technology and management of the business will be the extended arm of the dentist. Therefore, it's wise for the dental hygienist to add these skills to already perfected clinical skills.

Quality of Care and Teamwork

The relationship between profits and quality of service places many dentists in a desperate cycle, and lack of addressing dissatisfaction can spell disaster when you're the boss. Work environments that decrease quality of care and substitute quantity of patients to increase profits sacrifice work satisfaction, doctor/patient relationships, and professionalism. When time is limited for patients, it's also limited for training the team. When the choice is between patient and team, the dentist will choose to please the patient. It's understandable that the dentist places more stress on the team by wanting more production while providing less time for team members to enjoy learning and improve professionalism.

Balancing responsibilities is necessary for the office to function. Dental hygienists naturally take the lead for continuing education and life-saving cardiopulmonary resuscitation, or CPR. You can develop motivated resourceful management that can help the dentist in times of delegation of duties. Assume the leadership role in making sure the team is CPR certified and quarterly perform an emergency in the office to assure the dentist that the team is properly trained. Become CPR trained and certified to teach so you can instruct your team and other dental office teams in life-saving techniques.

Key factors causing demand for dental services include a steady growth in population and a growing population of educated consumers desiring quality dental care with a willingness to pay for these services. Be a promoter of your dentist and dental knowledge in the community. Nothing speaks more highly in marketing services than an educated, trusted employee who is knowledgeable.

The economy is always in fluctuation, but after 2009, higher rates of unemployment caused people to have less discretionary income to spend on dental and general healthcare. Private practice dental offices reduced personnel, but profit margins did not increase due to higher expenses in real estate. The real estate market in Texas was fairly stable, with Dallas and Houston leading the United States commercial real estate market. As rent, equipment maintenance, and team salaries increased beyond a normal 65 percent, this made the yearly compensation of the practice owner dip below 35 percent—the level most dentists prefer. The gross wages of employees are typically between 22 percent and 28 percent of total gross production.

Since team salaries can be manipulated downward in a poor economy, some dentists terminated long-term employees and used staffing agencies. These agencies prescreen employees, finding suitable matches, provide training to employees, and allow for a trial period of employment. However, keeping current employees who have exemplary clinical skills remains the best practice philosophy. Tenured employees know what's expected, are less likely to break an employer's trust, and develop a sense of ownership and responsibility for the practice. Overall, it's important for dentists to encourage team members to contribute to the practice. For example, front desk personnel trained in CPR can help ensure the safety of patients and support the clinical team in times of emergencies, increasing the professionalism of the office.

Leadership in Professional Dentistry

Organizations to which dentists and dental hygienists belong help define their professionalism. The American Dental Association (ADA) is specific about the role of the dentist as a leader. According to the ADA, "Pilot programs that test new workforce models should recognize the dentist as the leader of the team and be based on valid assessments of outcome, cost savings and efficiencies to increase capacity without jeopardizing the patients' health." It's therefore vital to the profession that dentists have leadership training, accept the leadership role, and have associates who are trained and accept the leadership role. These associates include dental hygienists.

Leadership means everything to a business. A person who can express clear goals and the mission of dentistry will set the standard of care for patients and model organizational behavior. Leadership engages the team by providing training and happier work environments. Building a culture of job fulfillment makes people happy. People who are happy positively affect the bottom line. My experiences over a 45-year span in dentistry indicate it's time for a surge of leadership training. Many dentists are slow to recognize employee dissatisfaction issues, and when they do, their attempts to address the problem focus on the wrong issues.

Dentists and dental hygienists are trained to provide services, and it's easy to assume other team members are in the office to help you provide the service. Every team member must be managed for satisfaction. Once an employee has decided to depart, the individual has little incentive to tell the soon-to-be-former employer the truth. Balancing engagement of employees is all the more reason to have measurable goals for each employee.

Continuing Education

Lack of communication is the number one reason most employees leave, and the process of hiring another employee should provide insight and a time for self-examination. Continuing education, or CE, hours are required yearly to retain license to practice in Texas. Specifically, Texas dentists need 12 CE hours yearly to retain their license, of which nine hours are clinical and three hours consist of an ethics course. Dental hygienists and dental assistants are required to take 15 CE hours to retain their license yearly.

Communication is vital for challenging issues. Clinical advances are constantly changing, and changes in education have required teachers to be trained in cultural sensitivity. Issues that include cultural sensitivity, disabilities, and workplace abuse require professionals to exhibit effective learning and behavioral change. If the dental hygienist develops and manages office systems and leads people, leadership training is essential. Developing leadership skills will produce leaders who communicate more effectively so harmony, continuous learning, and progress can be accomplished.

Patients become anxious with dental issues, and when dental hygienists are willing to unequivocally confront the major anxieties of dentistry, they display the essence of leadership.

Questions to Consider

- What are your suggestions to develop professionalism in dentistry?

- How can leadership be developed in the dental office or clinic?

- Should three continuing education hours of leadership training be required for all dental professionals to retain their license?

- As new technologies are developed, should dental supply companies that sell them require dental professionals to obtain continuing education and certification in mastering the technology?

- Should new technology competencies and skills be reported annually to retain or improve a dental hygiene license?

- Should cultural sensitivity and workplace safety courses be required for relicense to avoid workplace bullying and abuse?

- Should dental hygienists be required to become certified in ADA coding for the procedures performed by the hygienist and submitted to insurance?

- Should a dental hygienist as the provider be responsible for submission of a fraudulent insurance claim if billed under the dentist's provider number?

- Should dental hygienists have their own provider number when submitting a claim to insurance companies?

Recommendations

I urge you to become aware of issues that are commonly addressed by the State Board of Dental Examiners. Each month, cases involving dentists, dental hygienists, and dental assistants are brought before the board for examination. Some cases have poor outcomes of restorative care and may result in license revocation. Many involve integrity (or lack of it).

I would never want you to find yourself in front of the State Board of Dental Examiners explaining your decisions regarding patient care. If I had the choice of deciding one issue that might make the most difference in dental offices, it would be training in communication and sensitivity to understanding what factors enhance the working relationship.

Each and every individual can learn to be a leader or lead by discovering the control that lies within to make a difference and be ready when the need to lead comes.

CHAPTER 6: RISKY BEHAVIORS UNDERMINING PROFESSIONALISM

"You are the embodiment of the information you choose to accept and act upon. To change your circumstances you need to change your thinking and subsequent actions."

– Adlin Sinclair

What happens when a lack of ethical values from professionals in your practice becomes evident? For example, you may find the dentist's specialized skills exceptional but personal leadership values lacking. You'll need human connection, honesty, and transparency to have a good working relationship with your dentist. Everyone must embrace leadership in the dental office, but it takes courage to focus on areas in which you need to improve. No one can compensate for someone in the dental office who doesn't possess leadership skills. If anyone in the practice is struggling in this area, then implementing a strategy is necessary. As Albert Einstein said, "We should take care not to make the intellect our God. It has, of course, powerful muscles, but no personality. It cannot lead, it can only serve."

The word "leadership" means guiding others along a path and helping to define, choose, and carry out alternative choices. Typically, the dentist holds the vision for the office, while the hygienist and others direct the patients and resources with the goal of accepting and inspiring the vision. Hygienists coach their patients every day with dialogue that supports taking healthy, positive responsibility. The underlying message is trust mixed with an expectation that patients will "give it their best shot" to carry out the treatment plan. They respond to this leadership style and reciprocate with trust for the hygienist. The dentist and the hygienist, along with other coworkers, must form a team that has similar goals and values.

What does the dental hygienist listen for to assess and prevent problems in the workplace? For one, when coworkers suppress answers to questions and show no transparency, then look for social issues in the family. Usually everything else in the person's life falls apart before the job, but social issues can and do affect working relationships. You can certainly support solving these issues but not on work time. You can coach and empower coworkers to solve problems, keep a positive attitude, focus on the business goals, and move forward.

Also look for another deterrent to teamwork and goal setting—abuse of alcohol. People who ask the question "Am I drinking too much?" are being open about the issue. It's those who keep it a secret or won't answer questions about it who have a problem.

Keeping the wheels of progress going can be challenging at times. Be gentle with yourself and others, but if therapy is necessary for a coworker for any issues—alcoholism, drugs, improper sexual relationships, or any form of abuse—then set boundaries within the present environment or find employment in a more positive place. Because trust gets destroyed, problems won't be solved over-night and trust has to be rebuilt. Do your best to find positive ways for dealing with stress (e.g., exercise, involvement in charities). Accept these situations as opportunities for personal growth rather than let the challenges get you down.

Above all, learn resilience—the ability to recover from or adjust easily to misfortune or change—and grow emotionally from the bad experience. Embrace it first and then move on. Acceptance, knowledge, and the ability to recognize social problems in yourself and others is the essence of leadership. Establish and maintain a lifestyle that supports optimal health.

Standards of professional responsibility require both the dentist and the dental hygienist to create a safe work environment. A dental office can set up protocols that minimize risky behaviors that can inhibit the growth of the professionals. Successful leaders need awareness.

The following case studies describe dilemmas actually faced by hygienists in dental offices, told in a hypothetical way.

Case Study One

You have worked in this particular clinic for 22 years, I have worked here 20 years, and our other coworker has been here 10 years. As conscientious "board members" of the dental practice, we have to decide what to do about our wayward dentist and his "crush." The married 60-year-old dentist is involved in an extremely close relationship with a 25-year-old female marketing employee, LaRonda, hired to promote the practice.

For months, she and the dentist have been texting each other like a couple of school kids. Flirtatious, goofy, and inappropriate, he took a picture of himself at Men in Jeans Warehouse trying on jeans in the mirror. "I think you'll like these jeans!" he texted. LaRonda shared the photo and details of her recent raise with us—three conscientious coworkers—which made us feel uncomfortable. The dentist had never sent a photo of himself to anyone in the office, so why send this one to LaRonda? Why do we three coworkers have to endure these details? Even if the relationship wasn't romantic but just weird, it's still inappropriate. To work well, the culture of the dental office must be one in which team members feel comfortable.

In this case, the dental office is at risk financially. Performance has been poor for six quarters, and now the office is receiving negative publicity from people who refer to the office concerning the dentist and the person who was hired to help—LaRonda. General dentists who refer to this dental office question LaRonda's role in marketing. They wonder why they can't seem to talk to the specialist directly. As a result, this dental practice has become extremely vulnerable. Maybe it will all blow over, but we three coworkers are still uncomfortable when LaRonda is out marketing the office.

Our dentist used to be famous for his golden touch. He took a lot of risks, such as the procedure he did on Ms. Smith in which he rebuilt her mouth after oral cancer. In fact, his willingness to take risks turned his practice into one of the most productive dental offices around. His risks used to be exciting and fruitful, but now they seem harebrained to us. This relationship with LaRonda is just one more pointless, unnecessary, thoughtless, impulsive, destructive decision by the specialist. One risk too many. If his wife found out about this, maybe she could do something with him. A significant number of dentists who refer people to his practice feel the same way because they've made similar comments.

Plus, we worked better together before LaRonda came. Remember all the compliments we used to get from the referral dentists? But we haven't heard any compliments since LaRonda came to work here. Is it time for the three of us to prepare our résumés and leave?

Questions to Consider

- What effect does gossip have on the office?

- What concerns and suggestions can be presented to the dentist in this case, and who might be the best messenger?

- How involved should you get if you're one of the coworkers?

Recommendations

Gossip precludes us from finding solutions to the problem and adds a multitude of additional feelings among coworkers that could possibly lead to legal issues. Gossip lowers morale, increases anxiety among employees, causes divisiveness as individuals take sides, damages the organization's reputation, adds to lack of trust with employees, and jeopardizes chances for advancement.

As a leader, you will stop a conversation as it drifts toward rumor then redirect the discussion and avoid lost productivity. Alternatively, you'll let the person who is "gossiping" know this is unproductive and excuse yourself from the conversation. Others who hear these words will be relieved and you'll feel good that you've said "no" to something that wastes time and could cause harm.

Don't make the mistake of pretending not to know about the gossip or think that by admitting knowledge of the rumors you'll add credence to them. Instead, be attuned to the rumors and willing to take action. Solve the issue in a nonjudgmental, positive way.

Case Study Two

Jack and Jane were study mates in dental hygiene school. Five-hour energy drinks were part of the study regime, but a stronger medication, Adderall, seemed to help with important tests. Smart pills, as they were called, were shared by some of the dental students to relieve the anxiety of a test. What would it hurt to take one pill every once in a while?

Graduation came with no one the wiser. After school, Jack and Jane both found employment, and while Jack's life smoothed out, Jane's life continued to be stressful. After a hard day's work, Jane fell into the habit of taking a whiff of the nitrous oxide at work. She wasn't taking care of her body—not exercising, not eating correctly—and was in overall poor health. One of the side effects of nitrous oxide is the development of leg pains and numbness, called peripheral neuropathy, due to the depletion of vitamin B12 from using the drug.

Nitrous oxide abuse also causes numbness and tingling in finger-tips, with resulting loss of fine motor skills.

Peripheral neuropathy and mental confusion caused Jane to be terminated from her job. No one knew her issues except her friend Jack, who encouraged Jane to seek help. The lesson? Becoming addicted to nitrous oxide will likely end your career.

Questions to Consider

- Should Jane have been mentored at the beginning of employment to identify the stresses of the job?

- Does Jack have a professional or moral obligation to assist Jane or report her to the state board of dental examiners?

- What healthy ways can you list to decompress from a hard day at work?

Recommendations

In Texas, intake and assessment of drug violations can be submitted anonymously to the State Board of Dental Examiners. Cases are handled by the Professional Recovery Network (PRN), a confidential, non-coercive, non-punitive alternative to formal disciplinary action. The PRN program facilitates prevention, intervention, and rehabilitation for professionals who have (or are at risk for developing) disorders associated with functional impairment, suffering from chemical abuse or dependency.

The board's purpose is to make sure the professional is not a threat to the public. It provides long-term support for the professional to return to a productive place within his or her profession. Those who complete the PRN process successfully are able to correct behavioral problems.

Programs such as PRN help professionals adhere to a contract through a peer review board that reports to the State Board. Disciplinary action does little to intervene in the disease process and may frequently be counterproductive to identification and professional reintegration. By providing professionals an opportunity to enter into treatment and recover early in the disease process, the PRN can minimize negative impacts on the professionals, patients, and their families and friends.

Case Study Three

Dr. A and Dr. B recently merged their offices and decided to hire a dental hygienist. Tracy interviewed for the job with Dr. B and was hired for $38 an hour with a two-month probation period. She worked four days a week, nine hours each day, with a packed hygiene appointment schedule.

Tracy wanted to find out if she could get an advance on her paycheck because paychecks were paid only once a month. Dr. B was on vacation, which gave her an opportunity to talk with Dr. A. During the conversation, Dr. A stated he had observed her skill level and felt he couldn't afford $38 an hour; he could pay only $28 an hour. He said she could take the lower salary or leave. When Tracy told Dr. A this amount was well below the standard wage paid by most temporary employment agencies, Dr. A didn't respond.

Questions to Consider

- What would you do in this situation?

- Would you wait and have a conversation with Dr. B?

- Would you appeal to your employment agency?

Recommendations

When multiple doctors share an office, don't assume they share an equal business responsibility. A contract agreement between Dr. A and Dr. B may exist that indicates one dentist is less than a majority partner, and that dentist may have no right to terminate any employee. The bully boss may be the managing general partner and have the position to fire anyone over the objections of the other dentists. When accepting permanent employment, pose these questions: "Is an office manual available to read? Who is in charge of termination of employment?"

Ask to read the policy manual, which might indicate the procedure for conflict resolution and which dentist evaluates the conflict. If the manual commits to always using specific disciplinary procedures before firing someone, then the dentist is generally obligated to follow those procedures first. The time to understand the policies of the office is when you begin employment—before any misunderstanding occurs. When a conflict arises, you can hope the rules apply, but power is transferred in mysterious ways, especially between dentists.

Texas is a right-to-work state, which means the dentist or dentists in the office can terminate employment at any time and give no reason for termination. Most people think they know what rights they have at work, but frequently they're wrong. Workplace law isn't always intuitive, and just because someone is unkind doesn't make it illegal. For example, allowing bullying or acting like a jerk may reflect bad management, but it's not illegal. The exception is if your boss is being discriminatory to you because of your race, gender, or religion, in which case you do have legal protection.

Sadly, some dental offices are understaffed and economically challenged, and when people position for power, bullies like Dr. A do emerge. Currently, there is no federal or state law explicitly prohibiting workplace bullying. Many states are considering legislation that would make bullying conduct illegal, but even without workplace anti-bullying legislation, there is good reason for the dental industry to address bullying concerns in the workplace. First, if left unchecked, employees may assert claims related to bullying by sweeping the conduct into allegations of violation under existing laws. Second, if the conduct is prevalent and persistent, it clearly affects the workplace and the integrity of the dental profession itself. Until laws are passed, communication within dental societies, dental employment agencies, and the community seem to be the only ways to warn against bullies.

Incidentally, no state or federal law requires paid vacation time. Dentists offer paid vacation and sick days to be competitive and attract good employees, but a difference exists between what is wise and customary, and what is legal.

The connection between multiple dentists sharing office expenses is based on economics and the vision these doctors share. Guard yourself well; disingenuous visions for the business can entangle dentists and office workers, leading to a disastrous work environment.

For example, with multiple dentists in a corporate dental setting, one dentist can be the managing general partner and receive additional monies to administer the total practice. The other dentists either do not want to address business issues or only want to attend to patients. Overlooking the lead dentist's personal abuses of employees will only negatively affect the image of the practice. Beware that birds of a feather do flock together. With many dentists in the mix, it is extremely important to have rules and regulations.

Addressing the visions of multiple employers in a corporate dental practice is a relatively new philosophy for dental hygienists accustomed to working with one dentist. Issues with a solo dentist as boss get immediately addressed and solved, so this new paradigm requires employee finesse and professionalism at all times. Do your best to protect your professional reputation by having broad connections to community, organizations, and people outside of your work environment.

Case Study Four

Tina applied for a job with Dr. C and, for the first six months, loved the job. Her coworkers were delightful, but then she noticed that frequently one coworker would be fired and another person would be hired. This hiring and firing went on for one year and affected 30 employees. At that point, Tina didn't even bother learning the names of her coworkers. She no longer wanted to develop friendships with them only to see them fired.

Tina needed her job but was afraid to ask if Dr. C would be hiring a hygiene coordinator, thinking she might be the next person on the firing line. Dr. C suggested a hygiene coordinator be hired because Tina was constantly behind in record keeping and sterilization. Dr. C did support her suggestions for buying a Titan Ergonomic Scaler, selling Sonicare toothbrushes, and using a different fluoride varnish. Would he support other changes to the way she wanted to practice without firing her? She felt she was on shaky ground.

Question to Consider

- What performance issues can Tina manage?

- What analysis can she do to understand those issues?

- How would Tina feel about so many of her coworkers being fired?

- How could Tina explain to the dentist the impact constant retraining has on her performance?

- When would the best time be to approach the dentist?

- If you were Tina, what help would you want from associates in your study club?

Recommendations

Sterilization and record keeping continue to be two areas of conflict between dentist and dental hygienist. It's best to become informed of the duties through the Dental Practice Act and risk management rules. Hygienists are vulnerable in these areas, especially when it concerns oral cancer. Malpractice insurance companies such as Dentist's Advantage have been insuring dentists for more than 50 years (you can read archive case studies online). With oral cancer incidents on the rise, keeping good records by the hygienist is critical to avoid exposing the office to a legal issue. That way, presenting a change in patient care is made with knowledge and correct facts, reflecting the standard of care a hygienist is trained and licensed to do.

If you are in this situation, research various options, present your recommended change and its value to the practice, then teach others about the reason for the change. Team members, including the dentist, will observe and appreciate how you lead and teach by example.

Case Study Five

Dr. D is president-elect to the local dental society and will be slated for a position of leadership in the state dental association. That means he's absent from the office two days a week in service to these groups. One day a week, he devotes to administrative work for the local dental association, leaving only two days to run his office. When the hygienist first started work 10 years ago, Dr. D was in the office 220 days a year, but gradually, the hygienist has assumed more responsibility of the office while the dentist was away.

Over a six-month span, Dr. D's dental hygienist noticed he charged much higher oral prophylaxis fees for ethnically diverse populations. When she asked about his pricing policies for the procedures she performed, Dr. D fired her. Then, when future prospective employers telephoned Dr. D for a reference on the hygienist, he stated she "wasn't a good fit."

Questions to Consider

- How might the hygienist have reframed the question to ask about pricing policies?

- What knowledge has the hygienist gained for future employment?

- When involved with professional organizations, what communication should be addressed with team members by the dentist? By the hygienist?

- How many days a week is it appropriate for a dentist to be in the office to provide leadership, attend to the dental business, and maintain a dental hygiene department?

Recommendations

Management of time becomes critical when dentists provide leadership in professional societies. The added responsibilities directly affect the operation of their dental office and even their family life.

In this scenario, the more important recommendation is "don't assume." Coding issues are changing constantly. Because the dentist was involved in the organization, was he privy to information on coding changes that the hygienist didn't know? Did he present these changes to the hygienist? Has the hygienist attended a coding workshop in the past year? Coding workshops cover additions, revisions, and deletions that pertain to the dental industry. Courses offer advice for submitting efficient and clean claims.

From my experience, the coding for some dental procedures is subjective even between two dentists, especially if one dentist performs more invasive procedures. The term "upcoding" is used by insurance companies when procedures are coded as more complex than they are. It's difficult for two people to agree on a code when they have differing opinions.

In this case, the hygienist is correct in questioning the codes because "upcoding" a charge can be considered dental fraud. In Texas, codes the hygienist submits to insurance come under the doctor's identification number and therefore are the doctor's responsibility. To my knowledge, no hygienist has had a license revoked because of insurance fraud, but hygienists have been involved in offices where fraud has occurred and the dentist's license was revoked. As more current dental terminology (CDT) codes are added that relate to non-invasive hygiene procedures, hygienists will need to be informed to protect themselves from inadvertent fraudulent coding. Also, definitions of the dental codes associated with the dental procedures may need to be cross-coded to the related medical code.

To support the point, according to the Texas State Board of Dental Examiners, in the last 10 years with the economic downturn, no hygienist has had his or her license revoked, but 30 dentists have had to undergo this transition. That proves that dentistry needs non-clinical systems that improve the industry overall.

To have more than a superficial sense of how a complex entity works requires an in-depth appraisal. Dentists are influenced by consultants and the random path of successful peers. The best intentions of consultants cannot equal the effectiveness of the team when each member is "in the game" and accountable for results. The team intimately knows the workings of the organization and its patients. Often, the leader (the dentist) must step back and understand limitations, skills, aspirations, and goals.

I recommend performing internal practice audits. In these audits, the team looks at strengths and weaknesses, then commits each member to achieve specific results every day of the week and month of the year. This process avoids scapegoating the hygienist or any other team member. These audits help the dentist and team think through their situation. They provide a guideline to growth, development, and progress toward the goals set for the practice. As a team member, be sure to accept your assignments and study what's happening so you better understand all positions while gaining knowledge about coding and procedures.

CHAPTER 7: ADDRESSING ISSUES IN THE DENTAL INDUSTRY

"The society based on production is only productive, not creative."

– Albert Camus

Some practice management companies compare the productive dental office to the average dental office. "Take our course," they assert, "and your practice will be transformed from average to top producer." Marketing of the course might indicate that the average dentist works 175+ hours a month, takes two weeks of vacation, produces $400,000, and works 2,000 hours a year. The productive dentist works 100 hours a month, takes 10 weeks of vacation, produces $1,500,000, and works 1,200 hours a year. This justifies the consultant's fee when new figures presented at the end of the course reflect business progress.

Dentists who are in the office only 50 days a year will have a totally different definition of team-driven productivity than one working 220 days a year in the office. There is nothing wrong with solid growth year after year. In fact, this is sustainable and healthy growth.

Subtle but Destructive Power in Dentistry

Treatment plans presented by the hygienist are preventive in nature and easily understood by the patient. Patients are generally more trusting than they are of more expensive procedures, so they readily agree to a treatment plan that the hygienist presents. Interaction with the patient is cheerful, and the patient feels optimistic and more in control of a good outcome.

As a dental procedure becomes more invasive, people need more information that the procedure is worth the higher cost and will increase their quality of life. While the majority of general dentists refer to specialists that have their own separate office, another business model emerged when it involved surgery and sedation of the patient. This business model happens frequently in the procedure of extraction of third molars or wisdom teeth. Teeth extraction surgeries in the office are short; the dentist sedates the patient and performs the surgery. When a patient is intravenously sedated, the specialist is in control of the operation. This process performed by one person gives a sense of power to the professional because that person alone influences the outcome. Historian John Acton in 1887 expressed the essence of power well when he said, "Power tends to corrupt, and absolute power corrupts absolutely."

As a hygienist/office manager, I have personal experience with dentists who get creative when sharing office space. Power to control the outcome of where the patient goes for treatment frequently happens with general dentists and orthodontists looking to increase dollars in their offices on procedures they typically do not perform. Referral to a specialist involves the best care for the patient. When office space is rented out to itinerant "specialists," the dentist (and team members) convinces the patient that the procedure is safely performed. The procedure gets incorporated into office policy. This business model is responsible for patients not trusting the referral process because patients feel their well-being isn't a priority, but that the dentist and others in the office are motivated by profit.

How the general dentist wants to share his or her office space is left up to the discretion of the dentist, but the decision can be another indication of an inability to let go of power which plagues the whole profession. Whenever possible, it's best for the hygienist, office manager, and team to incorporate the sense of working together, sharing control and power, and helping everyone maintain a healthy humility.

Excessive need for control of power in an outcome causes continual trouble with team members and patients, and the distress can even be fatal to the provider. Of the five doctors I've known who committed suicide, three were oral surgeons, one was an emergency room physician, and one was a dental anesthesiologist. The last two had other risk factors that contributed, but the demise of the three oral surgeons was associated with an inability to control power. One wanted power over his body so he could continue to work after back surgery. Another wanted dismissal of legal action taken against him over the death of a patient resulting from complications of surgery. The third had the inability to admit that none of us is perfect.

I suggest developing relationships in the office that reject the use of excessive power. Know the warning signs. When challenging business decisions are made, have the courage to be an accountability partner. Leadership is developed by mutual respect for authority and sharing responsibility.

We all make mistakes, but we learn, and we must accept the complications.

Team Building

I suggest being gentle with yourself and your team during the learning process. Learning competencies takes a lot of practice. Take time to celebrate exemplary moments. It's important to display pictures in your office that support successes in your life because pictures prime your environment to prepare you for more success. They remind you to think in goal-related ways.

For example, I have photos of my family and places I have traveled on my office wall. When viewing my photos, I reinforce celebration every day. Plus, someone took the time to snap the photo so I'm reminded that any production, even a photograph, is produced by a team.

Do your best to ensure no one in the dental office is ever ridiculed, harassed, abused, or unnecessarily terminated, as these behaviors negatively affect team morale. Dentists who are extreme micromanagers want a team of employees who are robots and obey every command. This type of office setting doesn't promote team building, trust, self-efficacy, or respect.

Of course, the team must produce to pay the expenses, but production should not replace creativity or even curiosity. Curiosity keeps people engaged in their profession while engendering a desire to learn more and perform better. Pushing the team to produce doesn't promote generosity in the office to one another. It's necessary to trust and work well with the team to produce dentistry. No dentist or dental hygienist produces dentistry alone.

People's motives change and can affect work relationships. Just keep building a team spirit. Develop sensitivity but don't become sensitive. For example, a team member says something offensive to you, and you assume the person doesn't like you. What's the result? You either fight about the comment or you flee all future conversations. Both are unhealthy to the team because they deflect attention from the tasks everyone is working to accomplish. Communicate with the individual again to see if you get a better feeling or response. Asking the person's opinion on a different subject can get a better engagement. Don't assume the grumpy response is about you.

Cutting Corners

Whether it's a private or corporate practice, dentistry is a business that's governed by the profit motive. However, it's unethical and possibly illegal for a dentist to cut corners and sacrifice quality of patient care for the sake of quantity of patients to boost production. Although corporate dentistry receives unfavorable publicity when television news reports cases of Medicaid fraud, these issues also arise in private practice or public health clinics. To be fair to dentists, there can also be fraud directed at the business of the dentist by employees. According to the ADA, "the fourth quarter of 2012 survey indicated that economic confidence is down from the previous quarter. Dentist's economic confidence (DECS) index scores reflect dentists' feelings about their net income, gross billings, open appointment times, and treatment acceptance rates." Uncertainty brings out the best and worst in people, and that is why it takes a team.

Moral and Ethical Standards

Our own behavior is regulated by internalized moral standards that help us make comparisons, judgments, and decisions as we respond to various situations. When ethical standards are disengaged, however, people can be unethical without feeling guilty. The workplace provides ample opportunity to offload problems and diffuse responsibility.

For clarity and to create standards, the dental practice members can be trained as a team to identify risky behaviors. These may include (1) an excessive need for compensation, which may lead to a superiority complex; (2) inactivity, which may lead to apathy or depression; (3) escape, which may lead to drug and alcohol addictions; and (4) gossip, which keeps the team from achieving goals.

Having a clearly communicated policy that defines risky behaviors and self-contracts will alter your environment for the better. Being aware of clues will help avoid risky behaviors in the workplace. Continuing to complain is a natural response when feeling threatened. However, this strengthens the ego, which leads to taking things personally, adding to the conflict. Remember, you can always spend time more constructively by creatively thinking of solutions to the problems and ways to improve your life.

If a work situation is disturbing, you have the opportunity to take positive action and influence the people around you. Your goal is to help them be more protective of the work environment. Focus on solutions to problems that steal your attention, and then return to the small things that are easily missed in everyday life, such as smiles, compliments, words of gratitude, and honesty. You may wish to share with the dental community how you've solved various problems by writing a book or speaking about your accomplishments.

Training Hygienists to Administer Anesthesia

At this writing, Texas continues to deny trained hygienists the opportunity to perform local anesthesia, a decision contrary to all reason and common sense. Because of this, Texas-trained dental hygienists are experiencing diminished teaching opportunities at the universities. Directors of dental hygiene schools in Texas that hold multiple licenses in different states and are trained to administer local anesthesia are more competitive obtaining teaching positions. Therefore, Texas dental hygiene graduates have to go out of state to exercise the privilege of being educated on this expanded skill. Testimonies from dentists in states that allow this expanded duty of local anesthesia report better patient care and increased revenue.

Not allowing local anesthesia training has placed Texas-trained hygienists at a disadvantage because the bordering states of New Mexico, Oklahoma, and Louisiana do allow this privilege (along with the majority of other states). Lack of anesthesia privileges causes many hygienists in Texas to leave the clinical practice of the profession to acquire different skills and work in areas such as practice management, sales, or education.

Given that 45 states have successfully integrated the privilege, the question becomes, "What's the problem with Texas?" With more training, dental hygienists can be an even more valuable asset to the dental practice.

The Texas Dental Association has been the organizational voice of the opposition. Until private practice specialists such as periodontists or general dentists express the need for change, no progress will be made. However, decreased membership in these associations means less representation of the total industry's desires. It also means less discussion is given to expanded duties on a regular basis by non-board members who have personal experiences. When the economy is depressed as it has been, the majority of dentists are simply trying to make expenses, so the need for expanded hygienist duties is rarely addressed. Here's my belief: If Texas could historically establish the Women Airforce Service Pilots program, or WASP, the first women to fly American military aircraft in World War II, then Texas can train dental hygienists to perform local anesthesia.

I urge you to make the study of local anesthesia a priority, even if you have to go out of state to receive training. Prepare yourself for the anatomy training and attain peripheral knowledge so you can communicate more effectively with your dentist on this issue.

Other Possibilities

If a valued worker in the office becomes dissatisfied, the dentist might first ask the person if he or she would be willing to have additional training. If the dentist will share responsibility for training the team, then an opportunity comes up for dental hygienists to become training instructors. They can interact with other team members to learn new technologies and management skills.

I suggest you encourage your coworkers to continually improve their skills and set the bar higher to increase the full potential of the office team. The experience can provide the ingredients of transformational leadership. The goal is to retain good employees, especially if they've been employed a long time and their passion can be reignited.

Taking training classes can uncover issues that may not be easily communicated, such as medical problems with the employee. Fatigue caused by sleep problems, endocrine disorders, or being tired for whatever reason can distort problem-solving and decision-making abilities. An employee will need help focusing on work when worried about a sick child, life-threatening problems such as cancer, or a family member with Alzheimer's disease.

As hygienists, we work in environments with complex personal problems as well as complex technologies. Issues take time to resolve, but in the dental office, we are only as good as our previous day's performance. It's best to be supportive of all who have to somehow make it all work and show your gratitude for them.

People will continue to spiral downward if problems aren't resolved. At some point, therapy may be necessary, but professionals are reluctant to seek help because of their community connections. That said, sexual affairs, drug abuse, verbal and mental abuse in the office require therapy. Employees need to see a connection between work and the satisfaction of patients, or they simply won't find lasting fulfillment.

Employees need to know their work matters to someone. Feedback is necessary, especially when an employee demonstrates exemplary skill or positive work outcomes. Avoid employment with entities who constantly fail to demonstrate respect for the value women can bring as associates. If you find yourself in this type of practice, immediately look for another job.

Be fully aware that people have personal problems and they worry about those problems at work. Your dentist is no different. You need to think outside of the box at times. Encourage the resolution of issues through a mentor or training before therapy becomes necessary. Take the time to journal the day's activities. This is a coping skill that can release stress and aid with achievement of your goals.

Medicaid Fraud

Dental Medicaid fraud in Texas has been in the national news on a regular basis. These fraud cases involve hundreds of millions of dollars of taxpayer money and involve predominately male dentists, but two female dentists are also involved in one of the cases.

A dentist who's a lawyer and a past president of the ADA is at the time of this writing defending some of the allegedly *most egregious* Medicaid fraudsters in Texas Administration Hearings in Austin, Travis County. This is the worst time in the history of dentistry for fraud concerning dentist to dentist and dentist to patient that ever has been and I hope ever will be. Many of the alleged fraud cases center around coding misaligned teeth as "ectopically erupted" teeth to qualify the patient for Texas Medicaid orthodontic coverage. One of the accused dentists was on the Texas State Board of Dental Examiners from 2001 to 2008. Fraud and corruption are linked to workplace abuse, sexual misconduct by the dentist, verbal abuse, firing without reason, drug and alcohol abuse, divorce, and the list goes on and on.

In another case, investigation into the Texas State Board of Dental Examiners (TSBDE) reveals a female former executive director who resigned in the midst of alleged misconduct by the TSBDE. She was replaced by a male executive director, who openly stated the TSBDE has no authority to regulate corporate dentistry in Texas. This statement is in direct conflict to the federal circuit ruling (Fifth Circuit 07-30430), which is largely based on Texas statutes. In response, the Texas state legislature has passed new laws to better regulate corporate or multiple facility dental offices in Texas.

What does this mean to you? I suggest you avoid multiple facility dental offices and dentists who isolate themselves while trying to make a fast buck off of anyone they can. It will take every hygienist in Texas to understand coding procedures, teach and train about fraud, and report fraud in hostile environments. However, I believe in the heart of the hygienist to overcome and restore dentistry to its state of "do no harm."

"What's In It for Me?"

Texas needs to stop being a lawless state with lawless dentists who seem to do what they want out of greed. We need more examples of dentists who contribute to society rather than be convicted of fraud and imprisoned as felons. If this behavior continues, it will destroy the profession of dentistry and dental hygiene. In corporate dentistry, multiple dental offices, and maybe even in some solo dental offices, the question increasingly becomes "What's in it for me?" If this self-centeredness continues, standards of care will be diminished, not enhanced.

The ADA and ADHA need to address ethics because the professionals who pay their dues to these organizations need representation to eradicate fraud. Since dental professionals can't belong to a local organization without belonging to the ADA and ADHA, this corruption has to be addressed at the highest levels to avoid involvement with additional states. The profession will only continue to thrive if the organization protects the rights of individuals to work in a safe environment. Little progress against corruption will be accomplished by the ADA or dental industry if the ADHA doesn't form a partnership against this corruption. To do its job, the ADHA must address the issues of public safety as well as the well-being of dental hygienists employed in the industry.

Questions for Consideration

- How would you report fraud?

> - Do you think new laws giving regulators more power to investigate dentists performing unnecessary treatment will diminish the amount of fraud?
>
> - What are your ideas for solving the problem of fraud?

Recommendations

You can report dental fraud directly to the State Board of Dental Examiners anonymously. However, you need: the date the fraud was committed; the name and address of the dentist; the dentist's Medicaid number (if you know it); names and phone numbers of any witnesses; and a description of what happened. Examples of fraud include billing for services that weren't provided, misrepresenting services that were provided, and billing for covered services but performing cosmetic services. Other examples are double billing, altering records, and submitting a claim under one person's name when the work was done for someone else. Children are especially vulnerable. No one wants to be a part of an industry in which local news reporters investigate dentists who take advantage of children in a broken dental care system. When television programs such as Frontline and the Center for Public Integrity report on less-than-good dentistry performed in Texas, the public comes to mistrust the whole industry.

A New Way to Communicate Can Change the Culture

According to the U.S. Government's Bureau of Labor Statistics, the average age of a person in Texas is 33.6 years. However, both older and younger generations work in the dental industry. Even a few fathers and sons and mothers and daughters work together in the same dental office. The North Texas Commission confirms useful economic indicators, facts about the business climate, labor force statistics, and insight into the quality of life in the North Texas area where the median age is 34 years.

By nature, young people resist joining organizations. Apps for their phone help give them answers. Family and community have a different definition for them, and technology has been a big part of that difference. For them, email is obsolete, while texting is the way to exchange information. About 95 percent own a cell phone and 45 percent of those in younger generations receive television programs online. Most baby boomers still have a phone line in the house as well as a cell phone, and they place high value on the amount of work performed and belonging to professional organizations.

Younger generations want safe spaces to talk about issues without being judged, and blogging has been thought to be the perfect vehicle. Approximately 40 percent believe that blogging about workplace issues is acceptable. Blogging has become a suitable way to showcase accomplishments or recount the day's events as a way of decompressing.

Still, young dentists and dental hygienists want to make a difference in the world. Maybe the professional organizations need to listen and the dental culture needs to change. How can this new type of worker be drawn into professional organizations? These organizations must actually reach and interact with current members and prospective members to communicate that their membership enhances credibility for the profession. The viability of Texas dentistry requires increasing professional memberships and leadership from the next generation.

> ## Questions for Consideration
>
> - How do you think the dental organizations can best draw in and communicate with young members of the dental profession?
>
> - What new services would you suggest they offer?

Recommendations

Many organizations have developed multiple tier memberships. Some dental businesses operate primarily via electronic means; therefore, organizations are being encouraged to develop themselves in virtual ways. Younger professionals want access to up-to-date information in the field, professional development, and opportunities to network. With virtual organizations, members have greater levels of collaboration, cooperation, and information.

Virtual organizations could serve to reduce cost and problems of traveling to conventions. Video conferencing would allow professional organizations to broadcast technology to study clubs and schools and develop a strategy of getting the right knowledge to the right people at the right time. This would help professionals share and put information into action in ways that improve individual and team performance. In addition, virtual organizations would facilitate research developments in technology, products, and implementation at the members' convenience.

Case Study

You work for a dentist who employs many associate dentists in a multiple facility dental practice. The patient, a 16-year-old male, is not Medicaid eligible and can't afford a crown for a decayed molar tooth. As you walk by the treatment room, you notice the dentist is taking a paperclip, bending it, and cutting it with the drill. He picks it up and places the piece in the patient's mouth, then finishes the preparation while you are watching.

From your previous years as a dental assistant, you know that sterilized stainless steel posts are used when performing post-buildups following root canal procedures. Perplexed at why the dentist would use a paperclip when a box of steel posts is available, you continue to watch. You were taught in dental hygiene school that paperclips are not appropriate for use as posts. They haven't been tested for the mouth, they aren't sterile, and they don't have the tactile strength to undergo the forces of occlusion. Your next patient is being seated, so you don't have time to ask a question about the procedure.

You remember reading about a case on January 24, 2012, in which a former dentist pleaded guilty to Medicaid fraud charges. That dentist was also inserting pieces of paperclips into patients' mouths as posts in root canals instead of using standard posts made of stainless steel. The charges included assault and battery (two counts), larceny of more than $250 (three counts), a class C substance (one count), Medicaid false claims (five counts), tampering with evidence (one count), and intimidating a witness (one count).

Questions for Consideration

- In what ways could you communicate a challenge such as this in a work environment?

- How could you avoid being intimidated as a hygienist?

- How might you retain your employment while retaining your ethics?

- If after talking with the mother of the child, suppose the dentist agrees to a crown restoration instead of a pin buildup restoration. The crown will be fabricated by a dental lab that you know uses substandard materials. Would you inform the dentist of your findings on this dental lab?

- Would you inform the mother or patient of your findings concerning the dental lab?

- Suppose the dentist uses the substandard material, and the patient returns to the office for a six-month hygiene appointment. The tissue around the crown is bleeding, and the crown is fractured. What explanation would you give the dentist?

- Would your explanation to the patient be different?

- What obligation does the hygienist have to insure that the dentist uses reputable dental labs or product suppliers?

- What do the words "do no harm" to the patient mean?

Recommendations

I wanted to become a dental hygienist at a very young age. I had memories of a childhood experience with a dentist who drilled some fillings but didn't give me anesthesia. I was confident I could make dentistry a better experience. Everybody promises better service. Every member of the team represents great service; indifference should not be allowed. It's about dedication to excellence, and that prompts courteous care in which you're treated with grace and respect. You walk out feeling healthier and happier—and smiling more beautifully—than when you walked into the dental office.

I love it when dentists describe their abilities as "dedicated to excellence." Team members in the office and patients can instantly see the enthusiasm. It's a diplomatic way to work and demonstrates a mission of zero work stress. My favorite dentists state a position by asking, "What if . . . ?", "Would you help with . . . ?", or "Would it be helpful if . . . ?"

Questions allow problem solving and serve to solidify the team. Curiosity connects us to our profession and makes us exceptional clinicians. Hygienists take an oath that commits them to at *least* "do no harm," but the best clinicians maintain curiosity, which fosters enthusiasm to change lives. Curiosity sustains our interest in learning and continuing to study science as well as to apply that learning at work and with family, and to contribute as informed citizens.

CHAPTER 8: HOW TO IMPROVE THE CULTURE OF DENTISTRY TODAY

"Change the way you look at things and the things you look at change."

– Dr. Wayne W. Dyer

In the last 10 years, I believe dentistry has lost the vision of excellence. Ethical leaders no longer express how the practice needs to be managed. Corporate dentistry is a shared vision, and the idea of focusing on increased productivity alone has a way of compromising excellence in dentistry. The constant push for increased production, not the patient's oral health, has become the priority. Business incentives by an anxious dentist or practice management company often determine production levels, and procedure codes may be revised to include a charge for a procedure that wasn't done.

The dentist and dental hygienist need leadership skills to continue to place the patient first because *it's a privilege to serve.* Going forward, those in the dental profession must earn the trust and respect of patients, fellow workers, and the community every day.

I urge dentists and hygienists to create a goal—and exceed it—to ensure you have a creative but always compassionate professional environment, even though it may be challenging at times. Strive for continuous improvements, even if you have to paint your vision statement on the wall to remind yourself every day. Indeed, your patients will see the mission statement in your office and will appreciate knowing your values. The work is about trust and connection to the patient and all team members.

Look for clues to behavior in your coworkers that signal a call for support. Has the dentist or dental hygienist had a recent surgery?

Does the coworker need confidence to return to work? Perhaps the individual is too embarrassed to ask for help. How does someone who has just graduated and needs practice gain confidence?

If your life changes, find someone to explore new opportunities. Get support because issues that affect the dentist and dental hygienist affect the overall well-being of the office. Find the strength every day to meet the challenges, and when days get tough, remember the next day will be better. Mistakes made yesterday are in the past; this day is a new day. Know the qualities of a positive relationship. Watch how people respond to your positive news, and if they respond constructively, they will maximize the well-being of the environment. Surround yourself with people who are confident, have a positive spirit, maintain a desire to learn, and want to create a safe workplace.

If I could change dentistry, I would start with everyone being honest and transparent. Problems have a better chance to be solved when we can still smile, say thank you, compliment people, and be positive in our quest to serve our patients and coworkers every day.

A Coaching Culture

Coaching is designed to help facilitate professional and personal development for individual growth and improved performance with a focus on work or career issues. Coaching draws inspiration from disciplines such as sociology, psychology, positive adult development, and career counseling. Medicine is embracing the idea of coach training.

One way to find your way when you're unsure of making your goals is to hire a coach or develop a coaching culture. Coaching is a key factor in creating "healthy work environments" within a hospital setting. For example, physicians gain insight with coaching that allows them to assume the responsibilities of a hospital department chairperson or be on the board of directors. Trained nurses with experience in coaching facilitate many healing moments with patients and family members. Evidence-based research shows a coach is key to creating improved patient outcomes. Family members facing end-of-life decisions for loved ones can find true peace when unscheduled coaching moments are available. Coaching defuses many tense moments when emotions are running high and decisions have to be made in stressful situations that aren't ideal for making decisions.

Coaching would be valuable in the dental industry if a valued worker in the office needs confidence to improve skills. A coach could help the person discover the issues that need improvement and practice the skills. The issue can be simple or complex. It's beneficial to retain the employee, especially if the person has been employed long term and can learn the new skills. Coaching can also reveal issues within the office that may not be easily communicated.

To avoid office politics and secure confidentiality, hire an external coach rather than someone employed by the office. External coaches can be more objective and determine if the issues are resolvable.

Personality Assessments and Their Value

When hiring team members, some employer dentists are using assessments, or tests, that are supposed to predict if applicants are a good fit for the organization. Corporations have used assessments with success, but most businesses use these assessments for chief executive officers to determine leadership style. The tests are monitored by coaches who are certified to give the test and can give feedback on the results.

One of these tests, the Drive, Influence, Steadiness, and Compliance assessment (DISC) attempts to explain personality and behavior management style. The DISC includes an assessment that can be given to the dentist to determine leadership style. Emotional Intelligence (EI) refers to the ability to perceive, control, and evaluate emotions. Imagine a world where you couldn't un-derstand when a friend was feeling sad or when a coworker was angry. Psychologists refer to this ability as emotional intelligence, and some experts even suggest that it can be more important than IQ. If competition increases and employer dentists want to justify unrealistic production, more business consultants or employment agencies will promise dentists these tests can determine how to hire people that fit into the dental industry organization.

That said, *no* test predicts whether a dental hygienist or asso-ciate dentist will be successful at the job because those jobs involve clinical skills, and these tests predict personality and behavior styles. A few tests are available that determine decision-making and thinking styles. Many do a good job of identifying traits that can help an employer know if an associate dentist or dental hygienist is a good fit for the *camaraderie* of the practice. This determination could be positive for both applicant and employer because neither wants a bad fit.

Assessments might be used in the dental industry for self-awareness and personal and professional development rather than employee screening. If the employer dentist requires an assess-ment, the prospective employee or employee is advised to insist that the assessment be used only as a coaching assessment with a certified coach and not as grounds for hiring or termination. The results should be for the employee's benefit and self-efficacy. No one wants to risk not getting hired, but would you want to work for someone who doesn't respect an employee's rights?

Improving and Expanding Preventive Care

I would like to see every child in elementary school receive preven-tive dental treatment and education. These children would benefit by having improved dental health and some might choose the pro-fession of dentistry and dental hygiene as a result of exposure to a positive role model. The educational system could offer employment opportunities for dental hygienists similar to the school nurse program.

Expanding dental hygiene duties would help provide a partner for the dentist to help with access and provide appropriate care in underserved areas. This trend in many states has seen great success! For example, the State of Connecticut has expanded its dental hygiene programs to develop the job of advanced dental hygiene practitioner (ADHP). The ADHP is a state licensed dental hygiene professional who hold a master's degree in dental hygiene with established educational and expanded clinical competencies. In addition to providing oral care to patients, these professionals can work in hospitals, dental education, or dental research. ADHP training represents an important step in the development and maintenance of a robust and sustainable dental health care system while controlling costs. The hope is that ADHP training will aid in the efficiency of Connecticut's dental network much the same way advanced practice registered nurses and physician assistants have increased access to medical care and reduced the overall cost of care. It will take more than five years to determine the impact of ADHP programs, but the sooner the better. Physician assistants have been trained for over 40 years, and their importance to the field of medicine is just now gaining wide acceptance.

New Jersey allows certified hygienists to expand their practices under the supervision of a dentist to schools, clinics, nursing homes, hospitals, prisons, and facilities that treat individuals with developmental disabilities. Illinois legislators allow hygienists with certification in infection control and medical emergencies to work for health care facilities and perform hygiene services without requiring patients to first be examined by a dentist.

I would like for Texas dentistry to again focus on preventive dental care and dental treatment diagnosis. This would improve quality of life for the citizens of Texas and enhance the value of dentistry in the eyes of the public. To achieve that, hygienists require more training in oral pathology. Oral cancer education and prevention is critical to clinical hygiene education. I would like to see dental hygienists be invited to participate in oral surgery and oral pathology dental study clubs or even initiate a study club. A dental hygienist who understands how oral hygiene is related to systemic health becomes an essential team member with the dentist in the fight against cancer. I encourage dental hygienists to write articles on these topics and submit them for publication.

Another item on my wish list is for dental hygiene schools to help develop professional education programs in which students from different fields in health science could work together for a holistic approach to patient care. In Texas, dental hygiene schools are limited to 72 credit hours. Other states allow unlimited credit hours or maximums in the high 80s for an associate degree. The credit-hour limit hinders the educator's ability to add important subjects. Possible solutions might be to offer hygienists additional certifications in areas such as holistic medicine, working in nursing homes, and working in schools. This approach to education allows for additional training in oral health as it relates to systemic health, thus providing a broader base of knowledge for the licensed dental hygienist. Skill sets can be learned by professionals in dentistry, counseling, nursing, pharmacy, and public health that help them better reach unserved and underserved populations. Such additional education would also provide impetus for future training and research.

Building Bridges

Texas dental and dental hygiene state annual sessions for the governing bodies of each profession historically were held together. Then in the mid-1980s, dental hygienists developed a separate state session, not associated with one of the three largest dental conventions. We've educated thousands of hygiene students since the mid-1980s who haven't experienced joint state conventions.

The complexity of governing may explain the increase in dental specialty organizations with separate meetings and dues. Yet hygienists continue to work every day with dentists as a member of the team, not only as hygienists, but as office managers.

Despite additions such as the American Association of Dental Office Managers and Texas Dental Hygiene Educator's Association, a majority of practicing dentists and dental hygienists choose not to be members of any organization. Local meetings provide educational opportunities. Professions who work together want to learn together. Have so many choices of organizations contributed to diminishing relationships and more separation within the profession? Professional organizations must model team philosophy and leadership because that philosophy is vital to the industry.

In 2013, approximately 1,740 dental hygienists attended the TDA state convention to gain more training, many sitting side by side with their employer dentists. Besides the hygienists, there were about 2,850 dental assistants, 1,540 business assistants, 90 lab technicians, 575 students, and about 780 family members. They all prove dentistry is a team and sometimes a family business that supports the 2,560 dentists in attendance. With exhibitors, close to 12,000 people attended the yearly TDA convention held in May in San Antonio, Texas. The Southwest Dental Conference in Dallas attracts about 10,000 registrants. The Star of the South convention presented by the Greater Houston Dental Society is similarly attended, with each convention posting attendance on its respective website. The Dallas and Houston conventions have attendance by hygienists comparable to the TDA.

Texas is indeed lucky to have these three opportunities to obtain continuing education for hygienists in addition to the Texas Dental Hygienists' Association (TDHA) annual session in San Marcus, Texas. In times of economic downturn, money becomes limited for a TDHA session. If vendors and dental supply companies have reduced funds for conventions, companies could decide to fund only the national or state conventions and limit funds to a TDHA session not associated with a broader range of dental attendees. Dental hygienists could be the most vulnerable because continuing education is usually paid by the dentist when the dentist attends the same convention. Dentists rely on local conventions where information can be shared and new skills learned.

Enhancing the dental industry should be the mission of all professional dental organizations, and if the attendees come together with a desire to learn together, then the organizations would do well to improve and enhance team-building relationships. I'd like to see more opportunities for learning, teaching, and leadership that help mend rifts in the industry and inspire future dental professionals with optimism.

These are my dreams and I'm sure you have your own. Only by sharing those dreams will programs be started and progress be made to improve the culture of dentistry.

Questions for Consideration

- What can you do to improve the professional culture of dentistry?

- What does the future of dentistry look like for you?

- What are your interests in learning after dental hygiene school?

- How can you incorporate your interests and experience to help develop clinical certification for programs that can be taught in dental hygiene schools?

CHAPTER 9: DOES YOUR PRACTICE NEED A NEW PERSPECTIVE?

"The question is not what you look at, but what you see."

– Henry David Thoreau

Perceptions can limit us or inspire us. Behaviors are contagious, and when someone changes behavior, it becomes the norm. People then conform to the new norm, which is why it's so important to know your strengths and lead yourself.

To help themselves quit smoking, smokers make new friends who don't smoke, and these friends enforce a no-smoking rule. Connect yourself to positive people because they influence you in ways you don't even realize. Professionals who belong to study clubs or monthly learning groups have greater accountability and model appropriate feedback to one another.

This experience can transform a dental office. Working with other people to solve issues increases the base of knowledge, grows the professional's network, and gives the professional an accountability partner. Problems get solved in less time.

Positive Behavior Techniques

Whether you agree with the psychological influences or not, politics and businesses use positive behavior techniques. In politics, people are given pledge cards on issues and causes that involve cooperation. The words on the card express a commitment, and when people sign the card, they make themselves accountable. When it comes time to take action, they remember the pledge and act accordingly, whether it's voting for a candidate or giving money to a cause. Businesses apply positive behavior changes by teaching workers optimism. For example, when they log into the business computer, they see a picture of a coworker. The name of the person in the picture is the password, and this technique helps employees recall names during personal or business interactions. Positive behavior principles are being applied to certain spheres in life, and our perceptions are being changed by affirming the positive rather than denying the negative.

These techniques have been used extensively in orthodontic and pedodontic offices to promote acceptance. For example, a procedure is demonstrated using puppets before performing it on the child, and nonverbal communication such as a smile or a frown reinforces positive behavior and discourages negative behavior.

Working for a pedodontist is excellent training because smiles or handshakes become habitual, and rewards follow the demonstrated desired behavior. I suggest you know your strengths and lead yourself to the best life you can. I have changed my perceptions, and I have seen perceptions in other people change before my eyes. Here's an example from my own family.

Behavior Follows Perception

Tenth grade was just about to start for my son Todd. All summer, he didn't behave like his usual, happy self. Anyone who has a lively red-haired kid knows the mischievousness such a kid can display. I finally wore him down by asking him repeatedly what was wrong. He said he considered himself a disappointment to the family because of his decision to stop playing football.

He had internalized many not-so-truthful stories about men in our family playing high school and college football, and these had caused him to feel deeply anxious.

At the time, Todd was six feet tall and weighed 140 pounds. Standing beside him was his tiny mother trying to listen while wiping away the tears.

I reassured my son he would never disappoint me. I was proud he'd made this decision. I told him it was okay that his perceptions about playing football had changed, and he knew he had to move forward. Wisely, all on his own, he had changed what he believed, had made a thoughtful decision for himself, and had become a better man for it. What a powerful lesson I learned about understanding my child's perspective, and that moment would transform our relationship.

The best changes come from bold self-examination. Perceptions *perceived* are perceptions *believed.* Behavior follows perception. Thoughts are based on beliefs and how they're perceived. A new perspective is then conceived and usually stays in place for life. These perspectives affect every decision. So the moment you decide to change any of your perspectives is the moment you communicate and work differently. For a hygienist, working with a patient who is anxious of any dental procedure and then overcomes that fear to be a champion of dentistry is very rewarding. We want our clinical skills to be accepted and it's so rewarding to watch the patient, or even ourselves, get a light bulb moment and release the anxiety about a decision.

The Future Appeal of Dentistry

The profession of dental hygiene appeals to many because they get a chance to work closely with people on a face-to-face basis. They're responsible for creating positive outcomes in their patients' lives. Non-clinical skills (such as helping a person quit smoking) add value to that patient's health. However, there comes a time when the dentist needs to offer more clinical skills.

Just when hygienists think they have a routine mastered, the dentist wants them to learn how to use a new saliva testing device to improve perceived patient care. But they must perform this test within the same amount of clinical appointment time, which creates a challenge.

How do hygienists accept all the decisions from the dentist when they have concerns about implementation? How can they have confidence learning or explaining the importance of the new procedure to the patient? Hygienists are very protective of their patient's time to provide good oral hygiene care and prefer one hour appointment times with each patient.

Dentists in the past have developed more clinical skills as a way to fight it out in a competitive business. They turn to credentials from the Pankey Institute, Las Vegas Institute, and technology to set them apart from the competition. We live in an amazing age of dentistry in which everything is better and faster; but new systems and technology have to be converted to dollars that support the management side of the practice. They must also provide a standard of care that is paid for by the patient and considered "improved." Patients don't like to be coerced into treatment, and hygienists don't like to be a partner in selling coerced treatments.

Historically, hygienists have had little to no input in case acceptance presented by the dentist or input into the dentist's acquisitions of new technology. People understand why they need preventive services. Typically, hygienists have been that trusted individual with a steady stream of interaction with the patient. Dentists have tapped into that stream to provide opportunities for high-dollar case presentations with new clinical skills they are mastering. As dentists have realized that having more credentials or technological capabilities doesn't improve their case acceptance, they put pressure on the hygienist to produce more or sell more services.

Dentists want hygienists to help sell procedures. Improving the dentist's clinical skills—rather than changing non-clinical ways of doing business—has provided the easiest results in growth and sustainability of the practice. Hygienists are encouraged to produce more and sell more so more opportunity is available to the dentist.

Changes brought about by the dentist can be tough, especially when dentists consider themselves entrepreneurs. They take all the risk; they deserve all the rewards. Being an entrepreneur implies having more non-clinical skills involving qualities of leadership, initiative, and innovation in delivery or services. Team-building, leadership, and management ability are essential. The successful dental offices of the future will be those that offer a new model for working relationships based on collaboration and mutual value.

Qualities to Bring to the Practice

It's always best if change in management of the dental office or new delivery of services performed by the dental hygienist includes the following:

- Active listening
- Powerful questioning
- Communication
- Awareness of different strategies to aid in finding a solution to the problem
- Designing actions
- Goal setting
- Managing progress
- Accountability

When all of these aspects are involved, people's perceptions can change in a positive way—sometimes even the dentist's. Dentists are fact finders; they present logic to the patient and then the patient accepts the treatment. Still, acceptance of dental treatments is an emotional decision. Presenting more technology to the patient doesn't mean the patient will accept the treatment, can pay for it, or trusts the dentist to manage complicated procedures.

If you're a hygienist working under indirect supervision, I suggest you make sure the dentists you work with are transparent with communication. Try to understand the reasons for change and stay focused on your individual productivity. This will help reduce the times you're caught in a management issue that might involve termination of employment. In a power struggle, terminations usually have nothing to do with skill level, length of employment, or loyalty. Poorly managed transitions are unfortunate, and you may have no recourse except to move on to the next job. However, you can choose to look at the situation as an opportunity to find an office with a more positive, team-oriented perspective.

Dentists Need to Develop More Non-clinical Skills

The idea of expansion of clinical training that has worked in the past for dentists is being transferred to hygienists. But for the business model to grow, dentists need to develop more non-clinical skills. Developing non-clinical skills involve looking at business systems and deciding where they are today to get where they want to be tomorrow. The dentists that offer a new model for working relationships based on collaboration and mutual value will be successful, providing all this fits within the constraints of the Dental Practice Act.

The various specialties in dentistry are conducive to different personality styles, and transitions to working in different specialties can require adjustment for the hygienist. A pedodontist and oral surgeon have different ranges of procedures and ways to communicate to the patient and team. How the dentist responds to the patient during the procedure reinforces the personality style of the dentist. Does the personality style indicate the dentist would rather be in charge of all aspects of the procedure or does the dentist actively involve the hygienist in the treatment planning? Does this clinical style have any reflection on the business management of the practice? Does the management style involve the team? Exposure to different dental specialties allows for growth in your personal management style, also.

Being Well Prepared

Take time to develop a preparation worksheet that examines how you practice and create goals for yourself. Indicate to your dentist you understand the complexities of running a business, and you want to be involved in making changes that promote growth to the practice. Be a leader committed to doing your fair share. You want to be a team member who successfully promotes relationships and the productivity of the practice. You are accountable and you expect accountability. You are devoted to long-term success, and that success is related to putting systems in place that are beneficial and transparent to all.

Coaching and behavioral systems improve how you work and deliver care. Systems help you study risk of decisions, conquer false beliefs, and make the changes necessary to have a productive practice. If hygienists do nothing, they will get nothing. Build your system and share your system.

Here's hoping your future employment transitions bring joy, peace, and prosperity to your life, family, and work teams.

CHAPTER 10: THE LEGACY YOU WANT TO LEAVE

"Life is ten percent what you make it and ninety percent how you take it."

– Irving Berlin

Deciding how you want to practice is critical to your life and physical wellbeing. The choices you make and where and with whom you work determine your continued learning and financial, social, career, and community well-being.

Profit in dollars is temporary; but profit in a network of people—your patients and, collectively, the dental industry—who trust you as a person of integrity is forever. Every person who places trust in you will spread the word of that trust to at least a few associates, and word of your character will spread.

How do you know you want to work in a particular office if you haven't work there? You have to develop experiences, and the best way to decide what you like is to research the business and have the experience.

- Give every experience your full attention.

- Volunteer at nursing facilities and schools where dental health care is provided.

- Substitute for other hygienists or dentists on days they are on sick leave or vacation through employment agencies.

- Promote your integrity and intelligence at organization meetings, study clubs, and networking opportunities.

Birds of a Feather Flock Together

Inevitably, you become more like the people you surround yourself with each day. The dental hygiene profession is trusted by the public, and building a reputation as a person of integrity requires surrounding yourself with people of integrity. If you surround yourself with people who are willing to cut corners to get ahead, then you'll surely find yourself following a pattern of first enduring their behavior, then accepting their behavior. Develop criteria that are important in job selection, standards of care provided, management style of the practice, and the personalities of the other people in the office. Give every job experience a rating, with triple A being the best to single A being the worst. Be creative about opportunities in which you want to market your dental professional skills. Your word, conversation, act, and even presence can have a positive impact on a family member, neighbor, friend, patient, group, or community. Your legacy will develop, and with that development, you will be in contact with people who will inspire you.

Stories abound regarding less-than-successful employment opportunities with dentists who hire new graduates. Many employer dentists have forgotten how insecure they were when they graduated. Be gracious and know that everyone is in a particular stage of life. Know what you can produce without compromising ethics. Be familiar with business practices of area dentists when you go for a job interview and know how salary is formulated. Newly graduated dentists and dental hygienists need one to two years to develop skills that increase confidence. No one learns under intense pressure, so if a mature dentist hires a new graduate, the mature dentist had best evaluate, encourage, and take time to teach.

If you're a new graduate, know that confidence is built on transparency, so be honest with evaluation of your skill level and ask for help. Keep a dental skills diary and target questions that add to your improvement.

Journaling or telling the story of your life has been associated with a better immune system because you are healing yourself with words. You are making meaning of your life. This will help you achieve better skills because you put the past behind you so you can move on in setting and achieving new goals.

Tiers of Competency—A Model

Adult learning at the University of Texas at Dallas for advanced studies in organizational behavior focuses on teaching competencies. Competencies are knowledge, skills, and attitudes that affect one's performance on the job, which can be measured against standards and improved via training and development.

Every profession has competencies, but this program has three different tiers of training. Each tier includes different competencies. This model would work with any industry. A recent graduate would be at tier one and have three-month, six-month, and annual reviews. Conversational reviews and performance figures support the competency. Areas of improvement are identified and the employee gives strategies, so the review needs to be easily understood.

The employee can see how his or her performance is connected to the mission statement for the office and what is necessary to attain the next tier level. The opportunities for mentoring or coaching are an ever-present and enduring component of the work relationship. What will motivate the employee to attain the next tier is discussed. The employee can expect a negotiated percent increase in salary, depending on how close he or she is to reaching the next tier. Tier two has additional requirements, with final achievement at the top, or third tier.

Upon reaching the top tier, compensation is based on the local economy and the financial health of the practice. A compensation value can be determined for personal time off, pension plan, and additional perks such as education expenditures. A personal goal might be to finish a bachelor's or master's degree program, and if the employee is a top-tier producer, tuition could be a bonus benefit that the dental office provides. Similar to the hygienists, benefits can also be set up for the associate dentists that would allow for additional education to increase skill level. This is a fair and equitable way to ensure that compensation is appropriate for the skill level demonstrated.

Start Setting Your Legacy Now

I know a great dentist who practices on the east side of town, while most dentists want to practice on the west side of town. When I visit the office, the smell of the office is like fresh rain and I want to close my eyes and keep smelling. The music is soft in the office, with no television blasting for patients to view. The environment is one of trust and relaxation. The quality of dental treatment is exceptional, and patients are well satisfied with treatment because conversations are connected to the wellness of the patients that goes beyond their mouths. Not only do I want to keep coming back, I want to work there. As a hygienist, this is the mystique of the ideal office.

This dentist possesses a great knowledge of dentistry, medicine, psychology, and life experiences, and is well respected. The office and practice represent a powerful legacy of a calm and healing environment for patients. In fact, this peaceful atmosphere is the first comment people talk about when the dentist's name is mentioned in the community. The dentist demonstrates optimism, values, self-care, respect for others, good relationships, a sense of community, love of nature, and service. In other words, this dentist is a masterful teacher who not only inspires you but transforms you to give your best and improve your skills. When you come across such an individual, you count yourself lucky, because you know positive change is about to happen within yourself. No office is perfect, but it is these environments that create the impetus to solve problems. You are part of that equation, so study how you would make the office even better with your presence. Keeping this in mind will improve any environment.

One of my teachers in dental hygiene school is an icon. Yearly symposiums pay tribute to a passionate teacher for over 30 years, consultant to dental board examiners, and test constructor for the American Dental Association National Dental Hygiene Board. In addition, she earned a doctoral degree. With a ready smile for her students, Dr. Nancy Glick is a hygienist who has done it all and gives her all to the profession of teaching regardless of what life throws at her. As a source of encouragement to thousands of dental hygiene students, this teacher defines why our profession is so trusted and respected by her demonstration of impeccable clinical dental hygiene skills, integrity, and devotion to standards of care.

A legend is gathered in increments, in small steps, by a person who is open to change and learning new lessons, and someone who has grit. Usually, we have one special teacher in our lives who gives us hope. One teacher who empowers us to learn, welcomes us to the profession, and encourages us to find our way. An icon is not made in one month or one year. The years turn into a lifetime of making good choices, building on success, and learning from failure. Standards are set higher and higher, and one day a success is achieved and a legacy is built.

If you have that kind of teacher in school or at work, you have a role model that has inspired you to become a mentor or icon yourself. Leave your own legacy in dentistry.

Questions to Consider

- What characteristics have you observed in your teachers or mentors that inspire you to leave a legacy?

- How would you rate your present legacy?

- What are you not doing that, if you started doing, would be helpful in developing your legacy?

- When was the last time you did a self-audit to assess if you're on track with achieving your own legacy?

- How can you develop a roadmap of life?

- What areas do you need or would you like to have on your roadmap?

- How will you know when one of these areas needs attention?

A Toast to You

May you achieve your goals in the profession of dental hygiene and find your career rewarding. Passion for the profession will aid you in making many decisions at the crossroads of your journey. The dental hygiene profession is ideal for a mature, motivated, and goal-oriented person. Learn patience, persevere to pursue your passion, and be determined to succeed. Knowledge will add value to your career, and may it evolve in new and different ways to contribute to the optimum health of your patients.

A toast to you, and good luck with your career journey.

APPENDIX: GUIDELINES FOR DECIDING WHAT YOU WANT

Whether you're just starting out or wish to reevaluate your present career, the following categories and questions can guide you.

Questions to Ask Yourself

- What are your ideal job duties and your ideal practice?

- What employment opportunities have you experienced that were Triple A status?

- What skills are you good at that you never get to do in the practice of dental hygiene?

- What skills could you improve?

- What would you regret if you never had the chance to do it?

- What do you need to feel the happiest?

- What would add to your happiness? Examples might include: stimulating, challenging work, likable colleagues or dentist to work with, feeling that you are part of a team, flexibility, clear evidence that your work is respected, freedom to be more creative, feeling that you're making a contribution, opportunities to learn new things, rewarding friendships, helpful mentors.

- What tools would aid you in organization and promotion? Gaining new patients? Can these tools use or integrate practice management software?

- What mentors, coaches, and inspirational leaders affect your work and private life?

Short-Term Goals

- Personal
- Financial
- Athletic
- Health
- Hobbies
- Self-improvement
- Philanthropic
- Political
- Just for fun, I would like to . . .

Long-Term Goals

- Personal
- Financial
- Athletic
- Health
- Hobbies
- Self-improvement
- Philanthropic
- Political
- Just for fun, I would like to . . .

Factors That Promote Fairness

- Are you being paid what you're worth?

- Are you being given work assignments that use all your talents?

- Are you doing work commensurate with your abilities?

- Do you feel recognized for the full scope of your contribution?

- Are you doing your fair share of work?

- Are you progressing in your career at a brisk pace?

Identify Research That Can Aid in Factors of Fairness

- Mentors who might have encountered similar problems

- Professional publications/websites with articles that relate to your problem(s)

- Behavior norms for the people you work with and what their reaction to change might be

- Precedents or research for what you want to do differently

Questions to be Answered Before You Go to Work

- What is the mission statement and short- and long-term goals for the office?

- What are the dentist's and coworkers' interests outside of work?

- How do decisions get made on salary and purchases necessary for employment?

- How does the office engage in learning new procedures or changes?

Assess Your Bargaining Power

- Education

- Years of experience

- Special skills, unique strengths

- Work history

- Depth of knowledge or expertise

- Patient comments that testify to performance excellence

- Reputation in your field

- Calculations of average daily production

- Nonverbal behavior that will reinforce your cooperative approach

- Phrases that suggest a "let's work together" attitude

- Awards won

- Support of a powerful mentor

- Social or interpersonal skills

- Leadership or team-building abilities

- Knowledge of the dental office's culture, processes, history

Set Your Vision

- What is your vision for your future, your mission in life, your objectives and strategies for achieving goals, and your action plan?

- How is your vision plan similar to the vision plan of your employer dentist?

- If differences exist, what goals can merge to improve the dental office?

ABOUT THE AUTHOR

A popular speaker for dental hygiene schools, Deborah Lynn Malone Stewart is a dental hygienist, author, mentor, office manager, coach, consultant, and culture critic. With more than 45 years of experience in the dental industry, she encourages dental hygienists to continue their education and realize the impact of their profession.

Deborah advocates expanded duties for dental hygienists and business education for the dental industry. Although she believes it's important to join the ADHA, she also suggests new graduates become familiar with the Texas Oral Health Coalition. She notes that legislation in Texas will be vital to allow hygienists more autonomy and the ability to work more independently in public health. Deborah encourages increased education and advancing beyond challenges. She believes both are paramount for expanding skills and professionals must be students for life.

A graduate of the University of Houston with an MBA, Deborah also holds degrees in dental hygiene and organizational behavior and is a Professional Certified Coach (PCC). Her business leadership projects a proud and patriotic Texan. She's a member of The Daughters of the Republic of Texas, an historian, and a civic and community advocate.

Through her practical consulting and coaching efforts, Deborah helps clients maximize their abilities, develop the best strategy for team success, and manage reactions that may arise. Her collaborative, problem-solving approach propels them professionally and personally to reach agreements, achieve goals, ask for what they want, know why they want it, and get it ethically. She is a champion of both dental hygienists and the highest vision of the dental industry, in which she has played a significant role.

*****

You are invited to submit ideas or comments on the material in this book to Deborah at: **deborahlynn@me.com**

Connect through professional social network website LinkedIn at: **www.linkedin.com/in/dlynn**

www.ingramcontent.com/pod-product-compliance
Lightning Source LLC
Chambersburg PA
CBHW051318170526
45166CB00002B/590